Dietetics
Practice and Future Trends

Third Edition

Esther A. Winterfeldt, PhD
Professor Emeritus, Department of Nutritional Sciences
College of Human Environmental Sciences
Oklahoma State University
Stillwater, Oklahoma

Margaret L. Bogle, PhD, RD, LD
Lower Mississippi Delta Nutrition Intervention Research Initiative
Agriculture Research Service
United States Department of Agriculture
Little Rock, Arkansas

Lea L. Ebro, PhD
Professor Emeritus, Department of Nutritional Sciences
College of Human Environmental Sciences
Oklahoma State University
Stillwater, Oklahoma

JONES AND BARTLETT PUBLISHERS
Sudbury, Massachusetts
BOSTON   TORONTO   LONDON   SINGAPORE

World Headquarters
Jones and Bartlett Publishers
40 Tall Pine Drive
Sudbury, MA 01776
978-443-5000
info@jbpub.com
www.jbpub.com

Jones and Bartlett Publishers
Canada
6339 Ormindale Way
Mississauga, Ontario L5V 1J2
Canada

Jones and Bartlett Publishers
International
Barb House, Barb Mews
London W6 7PA
United Kingdom

Jones and Bartlett's books and products are available through most bookstores and online booksellers. To contact Jones and Bartlett Publishers directly, call 800-832-0034, fax 978-443-8000, or visit our website www.jbpub.com.

Substantial discounts on bulk quantities of Jones and Bartlett's publications are available to corporations, professional associations, and other qualified organizations. For details and specific discount information, contact the special sales department at Jones and Bartlett via the above contact information or send an email to specialsales@jbpub.com.

The authors, editor, and publisher have made every effort to provide accurate information. However, they are not responsible for errors, omissions, or for any outcomes related to the use of the contents of this book and take no responsibility for the use of the products and procedures described. Treatments and side effects described in this book may not be applicable to all people; likewise, some people may require a dose or experience a side effect that is not described herein. Drugs and medical devices are discussed that may have limited availability controlled by the Food and Drug Administration (FDA) for use only in a research study or clinical trial. Research, clinical practice, and government regulations often change the accepted standard in this field. When consideration is being given to use of any drug in the clinical setting, the health care provider or reader is responsible for determining FDA status of the drug, reading the package insert, and reviewing prescribing information for the most up-to-date recommendations on dose, precautions, and contraindications, and determining the appropriate usage for the product. This is especially important in the case of drugs that are new or seldom used.

Production Credits
Publisher, Higher Education: Cathleen Sether
Acquisitions Editor: Shoshanna Goldberg
Editorial Assistant: Teresa Reilly
Production Director: Amy Rose
Associate Production Editor: Julia Waugaman
Associate Marketing Manager: Jody Sullivan
V.P., Manufacturing and Inventory Control: Therese Connell
Cover and Title Page Design: Scott Moden
Cover Images: Woman shopping for produce © Yuri Arcurs/ShutterStock, Inc.;
        Oranges © Tihis/ShutterStock, Inc.
Composition: DataStream Content Solutions, LLC
Printing and Binding: Malloy Incorporated
Cover Printing: John Pow Company

Library of Congress Cataloging-in-Publication Data
Winterfeldt, Esther A.
    Dietetics : practice and future trends/Esther A. Winterfeldt, Margaret L. Bogle, Lea L. Ebro.—3rd ed.
        p. ; cm.
    Includes bibliographical references and index.
    ISBN 978-0-7637-7662-6 (alk. paper)
    1. Dietetics—Vocational guidance.   I. Bogle, Margaret L.   II. Ebro, Lea L.   III. Title.
    [DNLM: 1. Dietetics—trends.   2. Vocational Guidance.   WB 400 W788d 2011]
    RM217.W56 2011
    613.2023—dc22
                                                        2009045822

6048

Printed in the United States of America
14 13 12 11 10   10 9 8 7 6 5 4 3 2

Contents

Introduction ix

Part I   **The Profession** **1**

Chapter 1   **Introduction to the Profession of Dietetics** **3**

Introduction 4

The Early Practice of Dietetics 5

Founding of the American Dietetic Association 6

Influential Leaders 7

Dietetics as a Profession 8

Growth of the Profession and Historical Milestones 9

Reaching Out to the Public 15

Summary 16

Definitions 17

References 17

Chapter 2   **The American Dietetic Association** **19**

Introduction 20

The Strategic Plan 20

Membership Categories 21

Membership Benefits 22

Dietitian Salaries 22

Governance of the Association 24

Affiliated Units of the American
    Dietetic Association 31

Summary 32

Definitions 33

References 33

Part II   **Education and Professional Development** **35**

Chapter 3   **Educational Preparation in Dietetics** **37**
                  Introduction 38
                  Undergraduate Education 38
                  Program Requirements 38
                  Dietetics Education Requirements 39
                  Dietetics Education Programs 40
                  Trends in Dietetics Education 41
                  Supervised Practice in Dietetics: Dietetic Internship 43
                  Advanced-Level Education 44
                  Summary 48
                  Definitions 48
                  References 49

Chapter 4   **Credentialing of Dietetic Practitioners** **51**
                  Introduction 51
                  Development of Credentialing 53
                  Commission on Dietetic Registration (CDR) 54
                  Legal Regulation of Dietitians and Nutritionists ... 61
                  Summary 62
                  Definitions 63
                  References 63

Chapter 5   **The Dietetics Professional** **65**
                  Introduction 65
                  Scope of Practice and Standards of Practice 66
                  Ethical Practice 67
                  Lifelong Professional Development 69
                  Legal Basis of Practice 74
                  Evidence-Based Practice 75
                  Government Influence 77
                  Summary 78
                  Definitions 79
                  References 79

Part III	**Areas of Practice** **83**
Chapter 6	**The Dietitian in Clinical Practice** **85**
	Introduction 86
	Employment Settings of Clinical Dietitians 86
	Organization of Clinical Nutrition Services 88
	Responsibilities in Clinical Dietetics 90
	The Clinical Nutrition Service Team 94
	Clinical Dietetics Outlook 98
	Summary 100
	Definitions 101
	References 101

Chapter 7	**Management in Food and Nutrition Systems** ...**103**
	Introduction 104
	Areas of Employment 104
	Standards for Professional Performance 109
	Expanded Opportunities 112
	Summary 113
	Definitions 113
	References 114

Chapter 8	**The Community Nutrition Dietitian** **117**
	Introduction 117
	Community Nutrition Practice 118
	Public Health Nutrition 118
	Activities of Community Dietitians 120
	Career Paths 122
	Career Outlook 124
	Summary 125
	Definitions 125
	References 126

Chapter 9	**The Consultant in Health Care, Business,**
	and Private Practice **127**
	Introduction 128
	Becoming a Consultant 128
	The Consultant in Health Care and
	Extended Care 131

The Consultant in Business Practice 134
The Dietitian in Private Practice 135
Ethical and Legal Bases of Practice 139
Summary 140
Definitions 140
References 141

Chapter 10   **Career Choices in Business, Education,**
               and Health and Wellness **143**
Introduction 144
The Dietitian in Business and Communications . . . 144
The Dietitian in Health and Wellness Programs . . . 147
The Dietitian in Education and Research 154
Summary 160
Definitions 160
References 161

Part IV   **Roles Essential for Dietitians** **163**

Chapter 11   **The Dietitian as Manager and Leader** **165**
Introduction 166
Management and Leadership 167
Leadership 167
Management Functions 170
Skills and Abilities of Managers 173
Further Management Roles 182
Summary 182
Definitions 182
References 183

Chapter 12   **The Dietitian as Educator** **185**
Introduction 186
Educational Activities 187
Learning to Teach 187
Designing Instruction 189
Educator Roles 196
Types of Learning 204
Adults as Learners 205
Teaching Groups and Teams 206

Summary 207
Definitions 208
References 208

Chapter 13   **Research in Dietetics** **211**
Introduction 212
Importance of Research in Dietetics 212
ADA Research Philosophy 213
ADA Research Priorities 213
Research Applications 215
Career Opportunities in Research 217
Research Activities and Funding 220
Summary 220
Definitions 220
References 221

Part V   **The Future** **223**

Chapter 14   **The Future in Dietetics** **225**
Introduction 226
Changing Demographics 226
Trends and Issues .227
Changing Roles in the Healthcare System 235
Implications and Challenges for the Profession 236
Competition and Collaboration with
    Other Professions 239
Competencies of the Future Dietetics Professional . .240
Future Roles for the Profession 241
Summary 246
Definitions 246
References 247

Appendix A   **Code of Ethics for the Profession of Dietetics**
    and Process for Consideration of Ethics
    Issues (2009) **249**
Preamble 249
Application 250
Fundamental Principles 250

Appendix B   **Article II of the Bylaws of the American Dietetic Association** **253**
Members 253

Appendix C   **Headquarters Organization Chart** **257**

Appendix D   **Sub-Units of Dietetic Practice Groups and Member Interest Groups** **259**
Dietetic Practice Group Sub-Units 259
Member Interest Groups (MIGs) 2008–2009 261

Appendix E   **Position Paper Update for 2009** **263**
Food Choices 263
Food Supply 263
Life Span 264
Nutrition Management 265
Positions to Expire December 31, 2008 266
Position Papers Published in 2009 266

Index 269

Introduction

The purpose of this book about the profession of dietetics is to present an overview of the many career directions and opportunities open to dietitians. This is a time when the profession encourages students of today and tomorrow to take advantage of many unfolding career choices to explore and find professional pathways to a fulfilling and satisfying dietetics career.

The book is about the dietetic profession—what dietitians do, where they practice, and what is required to become a professional dietitian. Educational requirements and other data about dietetic technicians are also included. This is primarily a book for students: those beginning in dietetics, those who are undecided about a career choice, or those who are nearing the completion of their education and training and are exploring further possibilities. In addition, dietitians or others considering a career change will find information that encourages exploration along new paths of opportunity. In addition to career resources, information is included about education and experience requirements as well as credentialing and continuing education. Readers will also learn about the historical development of the profession, the American Dietetic Association as the governing body, and the future outlook for the profession.

Dietitians, through their unique knowledge of both the science and art of nutrition, are the professionals taking the lead in the promotion of nutritional public health. Because of this blend of scientific knowledge and the social and cultural factors that influence what people eat, dietitians are able to use their skills to help individuals in illness and disease prevention as well as those who are healthy and active. Dietitians also interact with professionals of other disciplines that affect nutrition and are able to blend their assorted expertise for the benefit of clients. Their participation in basic research and in integrating new scientific concepts into clinical and public or community nutrition practices adds an invaluable dimension to the dietetics profession.

Dietitians are prepared to be versatile through their education in the biologic and physical sciences, including nutrition, foods, food preparation and service, management, sociology, and psychology. This versatility of expertise of dietitians is especially critical as the international scene continues to expand, opening many opportunities in international nutrition, management, and food service.

Several changes have been made in this *Third Edition*. Strategic planning by the American Dietetic Association, newly revised education and experience requirements for membership and practice, a newly revised Code of Ethics, and updated results of membership and salary survey data have been added. Information on trends in the profession offering continually expanding opportunities for dietitians is emphasized throughout. Examples are informatics and the genetic basis of nutritional practice.

As in earlier editions, we thank the dietetic experts who contributed material to this book. Their valuable contributions are acknowledged as essential, especially the materials elucidating what dietitians do and how they practice.

We hope that students, teachers, advisors, and counselors will find the book informative and, hopefully, eye-opening regarding career choices. The authors believe this profession has much to offer students and dietitians of the future and attest that we have enjoyed satisfying and fulfilling careers in this profession. We hope that many who read this book will be inspired to become dietitians of the 21st century and will help create additional innovative career options.

Part I
The Profession

CHAPTER 1

Introduction to the Profession of Dietetics

**"An honorable past lies behind, a developing present
is with us, and a promising future lies before us."[1]**

OUTLINE

- Introduction
- The Early Practice of Dietetics
  - Cooking Schools
  - Hospital Dietetics
  - Clinics
  - The Military
- Founding of the American Dietetic Association
- Influential Leaders
- Dietetics as a Profession
- Growth of the Profession and Historical Milestones
  - Membership
  - Registration and Licensure
  - The ADA Foundation
  - Dietetic Technicians and Managers
  - Legislative Activity
  - Areas of Practice
  - Dietetic Practice Groups
  - Long-Range Planning
  - Professional Partnerships
- Reaching Out to the Public
- Summary

INTRODUCTION

"What is a dietitian?" "What does a dietitian do?"

Recognition of the dietitian as a food and nutrition expert became official in 1917. This, however, was not the actual beginning of the practice of dietetics. The use of diet in the treatment of disease was already an ancient practice even though it was based more on trial and error than on scientific knowledge. Besides physicians, others including home economists, nurses, and cooks were practicing and teaching about good dietary practices, and researchers were uncovering the secrets of nutrients in foods and their health-promoting effects.[2]

Dietetics has been practiced as long as people have been eating. The term derives from "dieto," meaning diet or food. According to earliest historical evidence, our ancestors were forced to concentrate on simply finding food with little concern about the variety or composition of that food. Today, however, food is plentiful. At least in the developed countries of the world, being able to choose and eat too much from that abundant food supply has become a major problem, resulting in adverse health for many.

Recommendations about eating and food choices have come from biblical admonitions as well as from early physicians and scientists. Physicians in Europe and China, including Hippocrates, formed theories about the relationship between food and the state of a person's health.[3] Many of the early physicians and scientists emphasized adding or eliminating certain foods from the diet according to disease symptoms although there was no knowledge at that time about nutrients. Until the discovery of the major nutrients in food during the 19th and 20th centuries, a scientific basis for many of the eating recommendations was tenuous at best.

During the 18th century, research by chemists and physicians began to yield information concerning digestion, respiration, and other metabolic functions. The studies were forerunners of later discoveries that identified the elusive substances in foods that were responsible for many of the effects described much earlier in the etiology of disease. Fats, carbohydrates, and amines were known by the mid-1800s, but vitamins and minerals were not discovered until the early 1900s.[4]

One of the most fascinating accounts of the relationship between specific foods and illness is found in Lind's *Treatise on Scurvy* written in 1753.[5] When it was discovered that lemons and limes or their juice would prevent the dreaded scurvy among sailors at sea for long periods of time, it was a lifesaving piece of knowledge. Vitamin C from citrus fruits was later termed the "antiscorbutic" vitamin. Other breakthroughs came when vitamin A was found to be a factor in the prevention of skin lesions and blindness in both animals and people, and when niacin, one of the B vitamin group, was found to prevent pellagra in humans and "black tongue" in dogs.[6] There are equally vivid accounts of discoveries of other nutrients.[7]

THE EARLY PRACTICE OF DIETETICS

Cooking Schools

Early cooking schools in the United States, following their emergence in Europe in the early 1800s, led the way toward good dietary practices.[8] One of the first was the New York Cooking Academy founded in 1876, soon followed by schools in Boston and Philadelphia.[9] The schools offered not only cooking instruction but conducted laboratories in chemistry and special classes for the sick.[10] The schools trained many of the men and women who were in charge of food service in hospitals and the Red Cross during World War I.

Hospital Dietetics

Early practitioners in dietetics were in hospitals feeding the sick. Because little was known about people's nutritional needs in either health or illness, food selection was not a major concern. Menus were monotonous and usually featured only a few foods. One account of menus in a New York hospital indicated that mush, molasses, and beer were served for breakfast and supper several days a week. Fruits and vegetables did not appear on menus until later, and then usually only as a garnish.[11]

Florence Nightingale is credited not only with improving nursing of the sick during the Crimean War in the mid-1800s, but also with improving the food supply and sanitary conditions in hospitals.[12]

Clinics

The Frances Stern Clinic in Boston was one of the leading food clinics established in the late 1800s to provide diets for the sick poor. This clinic continues as a leading treatment center and serves as a model for similar clinics throughout the United States.

The Military

Dietitians played important roles during the Civil War and World Wars I and II. During World War I, many served in military hospitals both overseas and in the United States. In World War II during the 1940s, hundreds of dietitians volunteered for active service. Dietitians also worked closely with the Office of the Surgeon General and the Red Cross to help train more individuals in nutrition. Military service and training programs are important professional opportunities for dietitians today.[13]

FOUNDING OF THE AMERICAN DIETETIC ASSOCIATION

The history of the profession of dietetics in the United States is also the history of the American Dietetic Association (ADA) because the two grew together in increasingly important ways. The profession flourished because the association took early steps to oversee both the education and practice of its members. In turn, dietitians supported the association and its activities.

Before the founding of the ADA, persons who worked in food and nutrition programs could join the American Home Economics Association (founded in 1909) and thus were able to associate and communicate with others of like interests. Dietitians were few in number and, although they had somewhat similar backgrounds, there was no way to identify persons who were professionally qualified. In 1917, a group of about 100 dietitians met in Cleveland, Ohio, for the purpose of "providing an opportunity for the dietitians of the country to come together and meet with the scientific research workers and to see that the feeding of as many people as possible be placed in the hands of women trained to feed them in the best manner known."[14] Because this was wartime, the government had extensive food conservation programs and used home economists, dietitians, and volunteers to conduct the programs. At the first meeting of the association, officers were elected and a constitution and bylaws were drawn up overnight. Dues were one dollar per year, and there were 39 charter members. Lulu Grace Graves was the first president, and Lenna Frances Cooper was the first vice president.

World War I was, in great part, the impetus that brought early dietitians together to discuss feeding needs. However, it was also recognized that the services of dietitians in hospitals were rapidly assuming greater importance, both in food service and in treating illness with diet. Researchers were making great strides in nutrition science and, as more became known about nutrients, maintaining good nutrition and treating certain illnesses with diet became more precise.

Four areas of practice in dietetics were identified: dieto-therapy, teaching, social welfare, and administration.[15] The vision of the early leaders is evident in that the same four areas of practice exist today, although terminology as well as practice in each area has undergone many changes. The first area, dieto-therapy, or the treatment of disease by diet, was later termed diet therapy, then clinical dietetics, and now is known as medical nutrition therapy or clinical nutrition. Dietitians in the practice of teaching instructed dietetics students, nurses, physicians, and patients. Later called the education section, this group established education standards and specified the experiences needed in an internship to become professionally competent. The social welfare area of practice was later named community nutrition. The administration practice became known as institution administration and later food systems management or management in food and nutrition.

The association continued to grow and by 1927 had 1200 members. The office headquarters were located in Chicago, and the association was legally incorporated in the State of Illinois. The first edition of the *Journal of the American Dietetic Association* was published in 1925, with four issues per year. Early issues of the journal featured subjects similar to those published today, such as articles on hospital food service, personnel issues, and special diets, especially the diabetic diet.

INFLUENTIAL LEADERS

Sarah Tyson Rorer has been credited as the first American dietitian. She was an instructor in one of the early cooking schools and educated both dietitians and physicians in hospital dietetics. Ellen H. Richards was the founder and leader of the home economics movement and so is claimed as one of the early leaders in dietetics. Lulu Graves served as the first president of the ADA and established a training course for hospital dietitians at Cornell University. Lenna Frances Cooper was an early ADA president and director of the School of Home Economics at Battle Creek Health Care Institution in Michigan. Later, she was appointed to the staff of the U.S. Surgeon General in Washington, D.C. She is commemorated through a lecture presented each year at the annual meeting of the ADA by a current leader in the profession.[16]

Ruth Wheeler prepared the first outline of a training course for student dietitians that established education requirements for dietetics practice. Mary E. Barber, another ADA president, was the director of home economics at Battle Creek and was appointed as a food consultant in 1941 to assist with the problems of feeding 1.5 million soldiers in World War II. She also edited the first official history of the ADA. Mary Schwartz Rose was a leader in nutrition research and nutrition education for the public and established the Department of Nutrition at Columbia University. The Mary Schwartz Rose Fellowship for graduate study is awarded yearly in honor of this outstanding scientist and scholar.[17]

Mary P. Huddleston was the editor of the ADA journal from 1927 to 1946. An annual award is presented in her name to the author of the best article published in the previous year's journal. Anna Boller Beach was the first executive secretary of the ADA in 1923, served as president, and was the historian of the association for many years. Lydia J. Roberts was a leading nutritionist at the University of Chicago and the University of Puerto Rico. She initiated nutrition education programs to improve the nutritional status of children in Puerto Rico and was recognized widely for this accomplishment. Mary deGarmo Bryan inspected hospital training courses for dietitians in the 1930s and also developed a training course for directors of school lunch programs.

Scores of other influential leaders led the way in dietetics. Additional information can be found in *Carry the Flame: The History of the American Dietetic Association*[18] and in the ADA journal. This brief listing highlights those leaders who played key roles in founding the association and thus were pioneers in the profession of dietetics.

DIETETICS AS A PROFESSION

A profession is defined as an area of practice with the following characteristics: specialized knowledge, continuing education, a code of ethics, and a commitment to service for others. Plato first described a profession as "the occupation . . . to which one devotes himself, a calling in which one professes to have acquired some special knowledge used by way of instruction, guidance, or advice to others, or of servicing them in some art."[19] Dietetics, like other professions that fit Plato's description, is organized around these principles in the following ways:

Specialized knowledge. The ADA set standards for education as early as 1919. At least 2 years of college was first recommended, which later became a 4-year requirement or a 2-year course for institutional managers. Courses for the bachelor's degree were specified and, later, hospital training of 6 months was added to the educational requirement. Subsequent education plans were introduced that continued to specify needed courses. In 1987, "Standards of Education" were established by which dietetics education focused more on the outcomes of the educational process. The ADA set up a review process that periodically updated educational requirements as the profession grew and matured. Dietitians and employers alike recognize the specialized knowledge required to practice in dietetics.

Continuing education. When dietetics was registered as an accredited profession in the 1960s, a requirement of 75 clock hours of continuing education each 5 years was initiated. The ADA recognized a wide number of educational events as meeting this requirement and gave credit accordingly. Continuing professional education is a well-established function of the ADA through the Center for Professional Education, which offers conferences, annual meeting events, and other opportunities.

A code of ethics. The ADA developed a code of ethics for its members in 1942.[20] The code was updated and expanded over the years, moving from the "Code of Professional Conduct" to the 2009 "Code of Ethics for the Profession of Dietetics and Process for Consideration of Ethics Issues." Published jointly by the ADA and the Commission on Dietetic Registration, it provides guidance to dietetic practitioners in their professional practice and conduct.[21] See Appendix A.

Service to others. The seal of the ADA carries the motto: "Quam Plurimis Prodesse," which translated means "benefit as many as possible." Dietitians recognize a professional commitment to help the public attain optimal health and quality of life through the practice of good nutritional habits. The organization reflects this imperative in all areas of practice.

GROWTH OF THE PROFESSION AND HISTORICAL MILESTONES

Membership

In 1917, the requirements for membership in the ADA were lenient in order to bring in as many practitioners as possible. Gradually, however, active membership became based on individuals having attained specified education and practical experience. Several categories of membership have been added over the years, and at present, the categories are: active, honorary, international, retired, and student members.[22]

Membership in the ADA has risen steadily over the years. The membership grew by about 1000 to 1500 each decade until a growth spurt in the late 1960s, with the addition of about 15,000 members between 1968 and 1978. In 2009, the membership stands at 70,000 of which 3 percent are men.[23]

Registration and Licensure

In 1969, the association established the system of national professional certification under which the dietitian was designated a "Registered Dietitian" (RD). The title carried legal status and denoted the professional who met the education and experience requirements to practice, in addition to participating in continuing professional education, thereby maintaining currency of practice. A national testing program was also developed to establish eligibility. Employers soon became familiar with the RD credential and began specifying it as a condition of employment. Today, 75 percent of all dietitians are registered.

Licensure of dietitians occurs in states in which state governments have passed legislation recognizing the profession and awarding state-level legal standing. At present, 46 states have enacted licensure laws for dietitians, many with details of practice allowed, while others promote the title of Registered Dietitian.[24]

The ADA Foundation

As the arm of the association with tax status identifying it as an educational and scientific nonprofit organization, the American Dietetic Association Foundation (ADAF) solicits and accepts monies donated for scholarships, research, and other designated projects. Several major studies have been funded by the foundation, and programs and lectureships at the annual meeting have been made possible through gifts and donations.

Dietetic Technicians and Managers

The Hospital, Institution, and Educational Food Service Society (HIEFSS) was formed in 1960 as an organization for food service supervisors. It was an independent society but closely tied to the ADA through membership standards as well as financial support. The name was later changed to the Association for Managers of Food Operations (AMFO), and the title for members became "food manager." Persons completing a voluntary certificate program have the title "certified food manager."

Dietetic technician programs require specific education and training, usually 2 years in a community college program of study. As with the RD, the technician member also can become registered by meeting the specified standards and passing an examination. He or she earns the title "Dietetic Technician, Registered."

Legislative Activity

Early participation in legislative activity began when dietitians promoted a bill to grant military rank to dietitians serving in World War I. In the 1940s and 1950s, legislative activity centered around setting standards for employment in the Veterans Administration, passage of the National School Lunch Act, and, in 1946, support of the Maternal and Child Health Bill. Signaling even more extensive efforts, the association changed its tax status in the 1960s to permit active lobbying and made its voice heard by establishing an office in Washington, D.C., and taking positions on national issues. A political action committee formed in 1980, through which ADA members donate funds and recognize legislators who promote legislation on behalf of food and nutrition issues. Each year, the ADA identifies key legislative issues for particular attention and activity by the Washington office and members. For 2008, the issue was healthcare reform with a significant white paper prepared by the Washington office with recommendations for Registered Dietitians in various areas of health care.[25]

Areas of Practice

The practice of dietetics was first structured around four areas in which dietitians were employed. These were: administration, clinical, community, and education. Little was documented about the number of dietitians working in each area until periodic membership surveys were initiated in the early 1980s. As shown in Table 1-1, clinical dietetics is the area in which the highest number of dietitians work. Although this initially designated hospital-related dietetics, the clinical dietetics category now includes acute inpatient, ambulatory, and long-term care. The number of dietitians working in food service administration has declined in recent years as more dietitians are now practicing in clinical settings, the community area, and in consultation and private practice.

Table 1-1. Primary Area of Practice by Dietitians (percent)

Practice Area	1993[1]	1995[2]	2002[3]	2005[4]	2007[5]	2009[6]
Clinical dietetics	45	45	54	54	55	56
Food and nutrition management	20	26	13	13	12	12
Community nutrition	14	15	11	11	11	11
Consultation/business	13	7	11	11	11	8
Education/research	8	7	6	7	6	7
Other			5	4	5	

Sources: 1. Bryk, J.A. and T.H. Kornblum. "Report on the 1993 Membership Database of the American Dietetic Association." *J Am Diet Assoc* 94(1994): 1433–1438.

2. Bryk, J.A. and T.H. Kornblum. "Report on the 1995 Membership Database of the American Dietetic Association." *J Am Diet Assoc* 97(1997): 197–203.

3. Rogers, D. "Report on the ADA 2002 Dietetics Compensation and Benefits Survey." *J Am Diet Assoc* 103(2003): 243–255.

4. Rogers, D. "Dietetics Salaries on the Rise." *J Am Diet Assoc* 106(2006): 296–305.

5. Rogers, D. "Compensation and Benefits Survey 2007: Above-Average Pay Gain Seen for Registered Dietitians." *J Am Diet Assoc* 108(2008): 416–425.

6. American Dietetic Association. Compensation and Benefits Survey of the Dietetics Profession 2009. www.eatright.org. Accessed October 20, 2009.

Dietetic Practice Groups

Dietetic practice groups (DPGs) are formed by ADA members practicing in or having a particular interest in an identified area of practice. DPGs provide a means of networking among group members. The groups elect officers, collect dues, and publish a newsletter or similar communication for its members. From the original 9 groups established in 1978, there are now 29 practice groups.[26] For a listing of these DPGs, see Chapter 2.

Long-Range Planning

Leaders in dietetics have consistently taken steps to position the profession to meet both present and future needs. This standard has been achieved through planning groups, task forces, committees, and outside consultants. In 1959, a study determined that active recruitment, educational opportunities, interaction with other professional groups, and an emphasis on research were needed for continued growth and development of the profession. These goals were expanded in the 1970s with the appointment of a task force and a study commission on dietetics. The study outcome was a report that examined the roles of dietitians and their educational needs for the future. The report, titled "The Profession of Dietetics: The Report of the Study Commission on Dietetics,"[27] influenced the ADA's direction for many years. A second in-depth study funded by the ADAF in 1984 became a major reference source for long-range planning.[28]

Many planning activities were initiated in the 1980s that moved the profession forward in significant ways. The first of a series of long-range planning conferences convened in 1981, with a second in 1984. Invited leaders discussed goals and needs and made far-reaching recommendations. The future was also explored in a strategic planning conference in 1995.[29] The ADA moved decisively toward public outreach and increased involvement in the policy arena, although emphasis continued on association members and their professional welfare.

Further landmark studies examined the education of dietitians, practice in dietetics registration and licensure, and advanced practice. In the 1970s a "Master Plan for Education and Practice" identified trends affecting the demand for dietitians and estimated numbers that would be needed in the future.[30] Role delineation studies included dietetic technicians and described the roles of dietitians and technicians in a variety of settings. These and other studies in the 1990s, including the Task Force on Critical Issues: Registration Eligibility and Licensure,[31] continued to show opportunities that enhanced both education and practice and led to continued advances in the profession.

Two task forces in early 2000, the Task Force on the Future Practice and Education and Phase 2, Future Practice and Education Task Force, initiated broad and comprehensive study of practice and education.[32]

The ADA Board of Directors undertakes long-range planning on a regular basis. Using expert consultants and the results of special studies and surveys, the board examines trends impacting dietetic practice to make long-term projections and set goals. The Strategic Plan of 2008 is the current document outlining the association's goals. The plan is discussed in more detail in Chapter 2.

Professional Partnerships

The ADA currently maintains liaisons with over 140 allied groups and associations. The formation of these partnerships has advanced mutual efforts and made many programs and activities possible.

Dietitians were initially organized as an interest section in the American Home Economics Association (now the American Association for Families and Consumer Sciences, or AAFCS), and joint efforts between the two groups have continued. The close association between the two groups is important in undergraduate education because most dietetics education programs are located in home economics divisions or university departments. Many members of each group hold membership in both associations.

Joint projects with the American Public Health Association (APHA) and the American Diabetes Association include the development of the diabetic exchange lists. Grants from the APHA also allowed the ADA to sponsor workshops on programmed learning. The U.S. Public Health Service (USPHS) sponsors a nutrition section that administers programs critical to health care in the United States.

The American Hospital Association is another important organization allied with the ADA. Hospitals employ many dietitians who contribute to patient care. Hospital-accrediting bodies (i.e., the Joint Commission of Accreditation of Healthcare Organization [JCAHO]) include nutrition and food services in their surveys and traditionally work with the ADA regarding the quality of the services. The American Diabetes Association exchanges speakers with the ADA at conferences and annual meetings and jointly publishes the booklet "Choose Your Foods: Exchange Lists for Diabetes."

The Food and Nutrition Science Alliance (FANSA) was formed in 1992 with the Institute of Food Technologists, the American Society for Clinical Nutrition, and the American Society for Nutritional Sciences. This linkage brings together a combined membership of more than 100,000 who have joined forces to speak with one voice on food and nutrition issues and to translate scientific information into practical advice for consumers.

The ADA has participated in many programs with governmental agencies, including the U.S. Department of Agriculture, the Department of Health and Human Services, the National Institutes of Health, the National Research Council, and the U.S. Congress. Dietitians have served on the Food and Nutrition Board to develop recommended dietary allowances, and on the Dietary Guidelines for Americans committee.[33]

The International Confederation of Dietetic Associations is composed of 34 national dietetic associations. The ADA was an early member of this group. The purpose of the confederation is to achieve integrated communication; promote an enhanced image for the profession; and increase awareness of standards of education, training, and practice in dietetics.

The American Overseas Dietetic Association (AODA) is affiliated with the ADA. The members are ADA members living overseas. The members enjoy the same benefits and privileges as other ADA affiliated groups.

An International Congress of Dietetics is held in a major city every 5 years. The first congress was held in Amsterdam in 1952, with the ADA as one of the founding groups. Organized for the purpose of sharing information, the congress publishes an international bulletin and holds an annual meeting. The 2008 congress was in Tokyo, Japan.

REACHING OUT TO THE PUBLIC

The ADA has initiated many programs over the years directed to the general public. Foremost among the services offered are the Web site: www.eatright.org and toll-free number (1-800-877-1600). The Web site is a source of current information for professionals as well as consumers interested in food and nutrition issues.

Begun as a "Dietitian's Week" observance in three states, this focus is now a month-long event each March with both local and national emphasis and known as National Nutrition Month. During the month of observance, media events, promotional material and advertising, and special programs are featured.

A "dial-a-dietitian" program, funded by the Nutrition Foundation, was started in Detroit in 1961. Many states now offer similar services designed to provide information in a timely manner in response to questions from the public.

A training program was initiated in 1982 to prepare selected dietitians to serve as spokespersons for the profession in order to reach the public with food and nutrition information through the media. More spokespersons, including state media persons, have been added in most major media in the United States. Referred to as the "spokesperson network," the program continues to be highly successful at reaching the public with timely and reliable information through television and other media outlets.

Position papers are another way the dietetics profession expresses views and presents "state-of-the-art" information in specific areas of dietetics. Before a position paper is published, it is extensively reviewed and approved as an official position of the association. Position papers are widely used and often quoted by the media and dietitians working to change or initiate legislation. Each paper is reviewed on a regular basis for currency of information to reflect the most scientifically accurate views.

Participation in national projects and campaigns is another way the association impacts the public. Over the years, campaigns on women's health, child nutrition, osteoporosis, high blood pressure, and other issues have been the focus of several medical and health-related groups, including the ADA. In 2009, the ADA collaborated with the Alliance for a Healthier Generation to focus on childhood obesity. The alliance is a joint initiative of the American Heart Association and the William J. Clinton Foundation and includes the Academy of Pediatrics, insurance companies, and major media outlets in the initiative on childhood obesity.[34] The national effort to improve the health of the U.S. population is centered in the National Institutes of Health "Healthy People 2010" campaign currently underway.[35] The campaign goals are updated every 10 years and include a broad range of U.S. health-related conditions and practices that require attention and improvement. In part because of the participation of professional groups and governmental agencies, this is a program with far-reaching implications for the public.

SUMMARY

The history of the dietetics profession is a rich account of consistent growth, forward-thinking leaders, and the emergence of dietitians as leaders among those concerned with the health and well-being of all citizens. As a profession, dietetics has established standards for practitioner education, a code of ethics, registration and licensure systems, and a tradition of partnership and collaboration with others in allied areas of professional practice to extend outreach and service. The ADA supports its members as they practice in a wide variety of careers, and also reaches out to the public with timely and reliable information about food and nutrition issues.

DEFINITIONS

The American Dietetic Association (ADA). The professional organization for dietitians.

The American Dietetic Association Foundation (ADAF). The arm of the ADA with tax status enabling acceptance of funds for designated purposes of benefit to the association and the public.

Dietetic Practice Group (DPG). An organized group of ADA members with similar interests in an area of practice or a particular subject area.

Dietetic Technician. A graduate of an approved dietetic technician program.

Dietitian. A professional who translates the science of food and nutrition to enhance the health and well-being of individuals and groups.

Licensed Dietitian (LD). A dietitian who has fulfilled the state credentialing requirements required to engage in the practice of dietetics.

Nutritionist. A professional with academic credentials in nutrition; he or she also may be a Registered Dietitian.

Professional. A person who has attained specialized knowledge and high standards of commitment in an area of practice.

Registered Dietitian (RD). A dietitian who has fulfilled the eligibility requirements of the Commission on Dietetic Registration.

REFERENCES

1. Barber, M.I. *History of the American Dietetic Association (1917–1959).* JB Lippincott Co.: Philadelphia; 1959, p. 3.
2. Corbett, F.R. "The Training of Dietitians for Hospitals." *J Home Ec* 1(1909): 62.
3. ADA. *A New Look at the Profession of Dietetics. Report of the 1984 Study Commission on Dietetics.* The American Dietetic Association: Chicago; 1985, p. 29.
4. Todhunter, E.N. "Development of Knowledge in Nutrition. I. Animal Experiments." *J Am Diet Assoc* 41(1962): 328–334.
5. Beeuwkes, A.M. "The Prevalence of Scurvy among Voyageurs to America 1493–1600." *J Am Diet Assoc* 24(1948): 300–303.
6. Goldberger, J. "Pellagra." *J Am Diet Assoc* 4(1929): 221–227.
7. McCoy, C.M. "Seven Centuries of Scientific Nutrition." *J Am Diet Assoc* 15(1939): 648–658.
8. Shircliffe, A. "American Schools of Cookery." *J Am Diet Assoc* 23(1947): 776–777.
9. See Note 3.
10. Rorer, S.T. "Early Dietetics." *J Am Diet Assoc* 10(1934): 289–295.

11. Cassell, J. *Carry the Flame: The History of the American Dietetic Association.* The American Dietetic Association: Chicago; 1990, p. 4.

12. Cooper, L.F. "Florence Nightingale's Contribution to Dietetics." *J Am Diet Assoc* 39(1954): 121–127.

13. Mathieu, J. "RDs in the Military." *J Am Diet Assoc* 108, no. 12(2008): 1984–1987.

14. See Note 11.

15. See Note 3.

16. See Note 11.

17. See Note 11. p. 161

18. Ibid.

19. See Note 5.

20. See Note 11. p. 131

21. American Dietetic Association/Commission on Dietetic Registration Code of Ethics for the Profession of Dietetics and Process for Consideration of Ethics Issues. *J Am Diet Assoc* 109, no. 8(2009): 1461–1467.

22. Bylaws of the American Dietetic Association. Amended June 2009, www.eatright. org (Accessed July 10, 2009).

23. Lipcomb, R. "2009 ADA Member Benefits Study." *J Am Diet Assoc* 109, no. 4 (2009): 596–599.

24. State License Information. www.eatright.org (Accessed October 27, 2009).

25. Health Care Reform Task Force Report. www.eatright.org (Accessed October 27, 2009).

26. ADA. "2008–2009 Dietetic Practice Groups." www.eatright.org (Accessed November 8, 2008).

27. ADA. *The Profession of Dietetics: the Report of the Study Commission on Dietetics.* The American Dietetic Association: Chicago; 1972, p. 2.

28. The American Dietetic Association Foundation Final Report: 1984. Study Commision on Dietetics: Summary on Recommendations. *J Am Diet Assoc* 84(1984): 1052–1063.

29. ADA. *ADA Annual Report, 1994–1995.* The American Dietetic Association: Chicago; 1995, p. 5.

30. Council on Educational Preparation. "Report of the Task Force on Competencies." *J Am Diet Assoc* 73(1978): 281.

31. ADA. *Report of the Critical Issues: Registration Eligibility and Licensure Task Force.* The American Dietetic Association: Chicago; 1992, p. 10.

32. ADA. Report of the Phase 2. Future Practice and Education Task Force. Chicago, IL: American Dietetic Association; 2008.

33. ADA. www.eatright.org (Accessed March 15, 2009).

34. Alliance for a Healthier Generation Expands Efforts to Combat Childhood Obesity with Launch of Landmark Healthcare Initiative. www.eatright.org (Accessed August 15, 2009).

35. Office of Disease Prevention and Health Promotion. U.S. Department of Health and Human Services, "Healthy People, 2010." www.healthypeople.gov (Accessed February 30, 2009).

CHAPTER 2

The American Dietetic Association

"In the history of the dietetics profession, there have never been more diverse or more interesting opportunities for dietitians and dietetic technicians. New levels of competence will continue to open doors in food and nutrition areas."[1]

OUTLINE

- Introduction
- The Strategic Plan
- Membership Categories
- Membership Benefits
- Dietitian Salaries
- Governance of the Association
  - Board of Directors (BOD)
  - House of Delegates (HOD)
  - Commission on Accreditation for Dietetics Education (CADE)
  - Commission on Dietetic Registration (CDR)
  - Dietetic Practice Groups (DPGs)
  - Position Papers
- Affiliated Units of the American Dietetic Association
  - State and District Associations
  - American Dietetic Association Foundation
  - Washington Office
- Summary

INTRODUCTION

The American Dietetic Association (ADA), formed by a small group of dietitians in 1917, stands as the professional organization of 70,000 food and nutrition experts. In the 90-plus years since its founding, the association has been the major forum for the networking of dietitians, presentation of research related to food and nutrition, and the political and managerial activities required to govern the large organization.

The original constitution and bylaws of the association have been amended frequently, but the focus of the association has remained constant from the beginning: maintain a concern for the continuing interests of dietitians and dietetic professionals in their education, practice opportunities, and research for the future. The ADA and the dietetics profession have become almost synonymous. The long-standing concerns of the two groups have consistently been the protection of the public in areas of nutritional health and disease prevention and the welfare of the practitioner (or individual member). The ADA and its leaders have worked through the years to keep these concerns in focus.

The mission statement of the ADA is "to empower members to be the nation's food and nutrition leaders." The mission statement sets the association's agenda and programs and clearly states the ADA's reason for being. The values that guide the organizational and member behavior are: customer focus, integrity, innovation, and social responsibility.[2] These values are defined as follows:

Customer focus—meet the needs and exceed the expectations of internal and external customers.

Integrity—act ethically, with accountability for life-long learning and commitment to excellence.

Innovation—embrace change through creativity and strategic thinking.

Social responsibility—make decisions with consideration for inclusivity as well as environmental, economic, and social implications.

The association's vision is to "optimize the nation's health through food and nutrition."

THE STRATEGIC PLAN

Development of the association's mission and vision statements, and the identification of its values and goals put a strategic plan for the association into effect. The goals help the organization's leaders to determine focus, set priorities, and assign resources in order to specify outcomes and establish what needs to be achieved. Three major goals are identified along with 16 strategies to help define how the goals are to be accomplished. The plan sets a course of action and the priorities for accomplishing the plan by 2012.[3] The three goals are: the public trusts and chooses Registered Dietitians as food and nutrition experts; the ADA improves the health of Americans; and members view the ADA as key to professional success.

In 2008, the ADA adopted a standard logo, replacing a mix of over 100 different visual brands.[4] The copy for the logo became: "Eatright. American Dietetic Association." The ADAF, the Pediatric Practice Group, and the Commission on Accreditation for Dietetics Education will use a variation of the same logo that displays their title.

MEMBERSHIP CATEGORIES

Membership in the ADA is available in one of the following categories: active, retired, student, honorary, and international (see Appendix B). The largest category is active, which generally includes those who hold a baccalaureate degree and have met the academic requirements specified by the ADA; an individual with an advanced degree and an emphasis in an area closely allied with dietetics; or a Dietetic Technician, Registered (DTR). In addition, any person who has completed a term as president of the association or has previously paid dues to obtain lifetime membership also may be considered as an active member.

The retired member category is an option for any member who is at least 62 years of age and either actively employed or no longer employed. Student members are those enrolled in an accredited program, a student in a college degree program intending to enter an accredited program, or active members returning to school for a degree in a dietetic-related course of study. Honorary membership is awarded to individuals who have made significant contributions to the field of nutrition or dietetics and are deemed eligible by the Board of Directors. International members are those persons who have completed formal training outside the United States and U.S. territories and have been verified by a country's professional dietetics association or regulatory body.

The rights and privileges of each of the membership categories appear in the bylaws of the ADA (see www.eatright.org). The dues may change from year to year by action of the House of Delegates. Those interested should review the current bylaws of the association for additional details.

Dues differ for each category, with a portion of the national dues offsetting the cost of the *Journal of the American Dietetic Association*, and a rebate returned to the state-affiliate association for each member from that state. In addition, the national dietetic practice groups (DPGs) charge for membership in their groups and provide newsletters and other educational materials for members in their specific practice areas.

MEMBERSHIP BENEFITS

Membership in the association benefits the individual and collective members in the following ways:[5]

- quality standards for entry-level education
- practice groups for networking in specific areas of practice
- evidence for positions on food and nutrition issues
- an annual meeting and exhibition showcasing the latest in relevant technology and products (the ADA Food and Nutrition Conference and Expo [FNCE])
- credentialing programs for various levels of practice
- a peer-reviewed journal issued monthly and a news magazine issued quarterly
- educational materials for continuing education and practice use
- access to professional education opportunities
- collaboration with international groups promoting global nutrition activities
- scholarships and research funding
- a code of ethics and standards of practice

DIETITIAN SALARIES

The salary levels of dietitians and dietetic technicians have risen over the years, with certain practice areas commanding higher salaries. These changes reflect the increasingly important roles played by dietitians and dietetic technicians. In 1938 it was reported that the hospital dietitian earned an annual salary in the range of $1090 to $7000. At that time, benefits such as room, board, and laundry were often supplied by the employer in addition to the salary. In positions other than those offered by hospitals, the salaries ranged from $1200 to $4000 per year. In 1946, the average salary was reported to be $3000—not a significant improvement.[6]

In 1981, the ADA initiated the first survey of members that reported salaries along with other data regarding employment. At that time, the average yearly salary was $16,400, although the study did not equate all salaries with full-time practice and the actual full-time salaries were probably higher.[7] The median yearly salary for dietitians in all areas of practice from 1997 through 2009 is shown in Table 2-1. In 2009, the median salary for all dietitions was $56,700. When all cash compensation was included the total was $58,000.

Comparing salaries by areas of practice in dietetics, it is apparent that dietitians in consultation and business have the highest incomes (median of $69,992) while those earning the least ($52,000) are in community nutrition practice. Several factors account for differences in compensation

Table 2-1. Median Income of Registered Dietitians by Area of Practice

Practice Area	1997[1]	1999[2]	2002[3]	2005[4]	2007[5]	2009[6]
Clinical dietetics	$35,491	$37,565	$42,825	$47,923	$51,668	$55,390
Food and nutrition management	44,924	48,924	55,000	60,008	64,002	67,995
Community nutrition	34,870	37,990	43,200	44,803	48,006	52,000
Consultation and business	46,040	48,810	60,000	53,768	60,008	69,992
Education and research	45,211	47,040	54,800	60,216	66,061	65,000
All areas	38,284	40,450	45,800	49,500	53,000	56,700

Sources: 1. Bryk, J.A. and T.K. Soto. "Report on the 1997 Membership Database of the American Dietetic Association." *J Am Diet Assoc* 99(1999): 102–107.

2. Bryk, J.A. and T.K. Soto. "Report on the 1999 Membership Database of the American Dietetic Association." *J Am Diet Assoc* 101(2001): 947–953.

3. Rogers, D. "Report on the American Dietetic Association Dietetics Compensation and Benefits Survey." *J Am Diet Assoc* 103(2003): 243–255.

4. Rogers, D. "Dietetics on the Rise." *J Am Diet Assoc* 106(2006): 296–305.

5. Rogers, D. "Compensation and Benefits Survey 2007: Above Average Pay Gains Seen for Registered Dietitians." *J Am Diet Assoc* 108(2008): 416–427.

6. American Dietetic Association. Compensation and Benefits Survey of the Dietetics Profession 2009. www.eatright.org. Accessed October 20, 2009.

levels, including years in a position, education level, job responsibilities, number of persons supervised, budget responsibility, and location.[8]

The median wage for the registered dietetic technician was $30,659 in 2002, $34,000 in 2005, $36,000 in 2007,[9] and $39,000 in 2009.[10]

GOVERNANCE OF THE ASSOCIATION

The organizational structure of the association has changed over time; however, generally the governance has been through members who are either elected, appointed, or volunteer from the membership-at-large. Those elected each year are officers serving on the Board of Directors, delegates to the House of Delegates (by state), members of the Commission on Dietetic Registration (CDR), and members of the Commission on Accreditation for Dietetics Education (CADE). Members of the ADAF are appointed, and membership in dietetic practice groups (DPGs) is by member choice. A chief executive officer (CEO) is employed by the board to oversee and manage a paid staff at the office headquarters in Chicago. Under the leadership of the CEO, the staff members form partnerships with the various volunteer groups, forming teams to accomplish the variety of tasks necessary to keep the organization functional and to implement the strategic plan. (See Appendix C for the organization of the headquarters office.) The Board of Directors (BOD) and the House of Delegates (HOD) function as a voice for members. Figure 2-1 is a depiction of the governing units of the ADA and their relationship with members.

Board of Directors (BOD)

The BOD is composed of 18 members: president, president-elect, past president, treasurer, treasurer-elect, 3 directors at large, 6 HOD directors, 2 public members, the ADAF chair, and the CEO of ADA, who is non-voting. The BOD governs the organization through the following activities:

- sets and monitors strategic direction
- oversees fiscal planning
- provides leadership for professional initiatives
- selects, supports, and assesses the CEO and conducts an annual performance appraisal
- appoints persons to represent the association

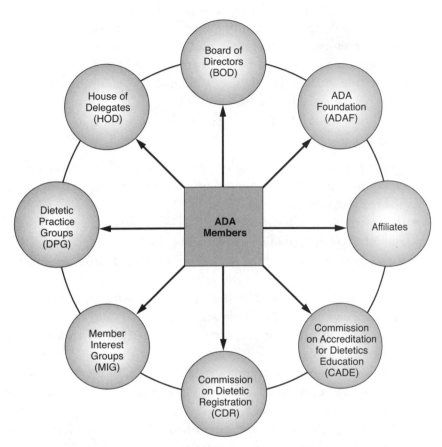

FIGURE 2-1. ADA Organization Units.

- establishes guidelines and policies for appeal, publications, awards, and honors
- administers and enforces the professional code of ethics
- exercises powers and performs lawful acts under the Illinois Not-for-Profit Corporation Act

House of Delegates (HOD)

The HOD is composed of 110 affiliate delegates representing the 53 affiliate (state) dietetic associations and elected by the affiliate members. In addition, there are 18 "professional issues" delegates representing the DPGs who are elected by the general ADA membership. Ten at-large delegates are also in the House, representing groups as follows: one delegate from the CADE, one delegate representing the CDR, two dietetic technicians, one student member representative, one retired member representative, one representing member under 30 years of age, and three delegates from the membership at large. Finally, six HOD directors comprise the House leadership team elected by the BOD.

The HOD has the following responsibilities toward governing the profession:

- partners with the CDR to adopt and revise a code of ethics for dietetic practitioners, disciplinary procedures for unethical conduct, and reinstatement conditions
- makes recommendations to the CDR on standards, qualifications, and other issues related to credentialing
- makes recommendations to the CADE on accreditation and related issues
- provides direction for quality management in dietetic practice
- identifies and develops position statements
- assists with recruitment and retention efforts related to leadership development
- establishes and maintains professional standards of the membership
- identifies and prioritizes trends and recommends policy and strategic direction for the association
- establishes qualifications and dues of members and the formula for dues payment to affiliated organizations

Both the BOD and HOD represent the ADA members and govern the profession. As a comparison, the BOD is likened to the executive branch and the HOD the legislative branch. Both groups work together closely to promote the interests of the members and to further the profession.

Commission on Accreditation for Dietetics Education (CADE)

The CADE establishes and enforces standards for the educational preparation of dietetics professionals and recognized dietetics education programs. The CADE administers and has authority for all actions that apply to accreditation of entry-level education programs, including standard setting, fees, finances, and administration. There are 12 members on the commission. At least half of the members represent each program type (dietetic technician, didactic, coordinated, and dietetic internship). The commission includes one representative of other constituents, a dietetic student, and two representatives of the public.

Commission on Dietetic Registration (CDR)

The mission of CDR is to protect the public through credentialing and assessment procedures that assure the competence of Registered Dietitians and Dietetic Technicians, Registered.

The CDR sets the standards for certification and recertification, and enforces the code of ethics of the association. The commission issues credentials to those individuals who meet the standards. Dietitians thus attain the Registered Dietitian designation and the DTR. Specialists receive the certified specialist title (see Chapter 4).

Dietetic Practice Groups (DPGs)

Practice groups are professional interest groups within the ADA framework. The 29 currently active groups show the diversity of the practice areas in which dietitians work (Table 2-2). Each group networks to serve its members, charges fees to support its activities, and publishes periodic newsletters. The groups also sponsor educational sessions at the annual meeting of the ADA. The requirement to join a DPG is ADA membership and the payment of dues. A member may belong to as many DPGs as desired.

Formation of new DPGs occurs after interest groups become large enough to seek official status. A petition is submitted with no less than 500 signatures indicating interest, a list of individuals willing to serve as officers, and a budget. Aside from maintaining a minimum of 300 members, other uniform requirements include publication of a quarterly member newsletter, maintaining governing documents, conducting an annual member meeting, and maintaining a budget. DPGs offer networking opportunities for professionals with similar interests and provide significant opportunities for leadership responsibilities within both the DPG and the greater association.

A DPG may also develop sub-units, or groups of members within the DPG, based on practice area or issue of interest to the members of the group, thus creating an even smaller group of dietitians with closely allied interests. Currently, 30 sub-specialty areas exist within the main DPGs (see Appendix D). In addition, Member Interest Groups (MIGs) have been

Table 2-2. 2009–2010 Dietetic Practice Groups

Behavioral Health Nutrition DPG	Impact the nutrition of the behavioral health populations we serve.
Clinical Nutrition Management DPG	Managers who direct clinical nutrition programs across the continuum of care.
Diabetes Care and Education (DCE) DPG	Members involved in patient and professional education as well as research for the management of diabetes mellitus.
Dietetic Educators of Practitioners (DEP) DPG	Educators of dietetic practitioners for entry and advanced levels of dietetics practice.
Dietetic Technicians in Practice DPG	Dietetic Technicians, Registered, dietetic technician educators, and others who are interested in Dietetic Technician, Registered practice and issues that directly affect the Dietetic Technician, Registered.
Dietetics in Health Care Communities DPG (formerly CD-HCF DPG)	Practitioners typically employed under contract who provide nutrition consultation to acute and long-term-care facilities, home care companies, healthcare agencies, and the food service industry.
Dietitians in Business and Communications (DBC) DPG	Food and nutrition professionals who are working for or consulting with local or global corporations, businesses, or organizations in food, nutrition, communications, public relations, and healthcare industries, or who are self-employed or business owners.
Dietitians in Integrative and Functional Medicine (DIFM) DPG	Members interested in the study of holistic, integrative, and functional medicine therapies.
Dietitians in Nutrition Support (DNS) DPG	Dietitians who integrate the science and practice of enteral and parenteral nutrition in order to provide appropriate nutrition support therapy to individuals encompassing adults, pediatrics, inpatients, outpatients, home care, and transplantation.
Food and Culinary Professionals DPG	Members who promote food education and culinary skills to enhance quality of life and health of the public.
Healthy Aging DPG	Practitioners who provide and manage nutrition programs and services to older adults in a variety of settings—community, home, healthcare facilities, and education and research facilities.

(continues)

Table 2-2. 2009–2010 Dietetic Practice Groups *(continued)*

Hunger and Environmental Nutrition DPG	HEN DPG members optimize the nation's health by promoting access to nutritious food and clean water from a secure and sustainable food system.
Infectious Diseases Nutrition DPG	Members sharing cutting-edge information on nutrition management of infectious diseases and providing an avenue for research, monitoring, and advocacy for nutrition intervention.
Management in Food and Nutrition Systems DPG	Food and nutrition care leaders generally employed in institutions, colleges, and universities; includes directors of departments of facilities and administrative dietitians and technicians.
Medical Nutrition Practice Group DPG	MNPG's mission is to empower members to be the recognized leaders who provide exemplary nutrition care.
Nutrition Education for the Public (NEP) DPG	Practitioners involved in the design, implementation, and evaluation of nutrition education programs for target populations.
Nutrition Educators of Health Professionals (NEHP) DPG	Members involved in education and communication with physicians, nurses, dentists, and other healthcare professionals.
Nutrition Entrepreneurs (NE) DPG *"Experts in the Business of Nutrition"*	NE members are shaping the future of dietetics by pursuing innovative and creative ways of providing nutrition products and services to consumers, industry, media, and businesses. Our mission is to help members achieve their professional and financial potential by providing the tools to build and maintain a successful nutrition-related business.
Oncology Nutrition DPG	Members involved in the care of cancer patients, cancer prevention, and research.
Pediatric Nutrition DPG	Practitioners who provide nutrition services for the pediatric population in a wide variety of settings.
Public Health/ Community Nutrition DPG	Members who provide nutrition services to all age groups in a community setting.

(continues)

Table 2-2. 2009–2010 Dietetic Practice Groups *(continued)*

Renal Dietitians DPG	A professional organization that focuses on chronic kidney disease and provides educational materials and resources for both professionals and patients/clients. RPG offers resources for both practicing dietitians changing their clinical focus to renal nutrition as well as cutting edge resources and advanced topics for clinicians that have been practicing renal nutrition for many years.
Research DPG	Members propose, assist with, complete, manage, and disseminate research projects conducted in clinical, community, healthcare, laboratory, and academic settings.
School Nutrition Services DPG	School food service directors and nutrition educators employed in child nutrition programs, and corporate dietitians working in companies supplying products or services to school food service operations.
Sports, Cardiovascular, and Wellness Nutrition DPG	Members with expertise in promoting healthy, active lifestyles through excellence in nutrition for sports performance, cardiovascular health, wellness, and the prevention and treatment of disordered eating.
Vegetarian Nutrition DPG	Members in community, clinical, education, or food service settings who wish to learn about plant-based diets and provide support to individuals following a vegetarian lifestyle.
Weight Management DPG	The Weight Management DPG supports the highest level of professional practice in the prevention and treatment of overweight and obesity throughout the life cycle.
Women's Health DPG	Practitioners addressing women's health and nutrition care issues throughout the life cycle.

Source: Courtesy of the American Dietetic Association.

formed whereby specific population groups can share mutual interests (see Appendix D).

Position Papers

A position paper represents a consensus of viewpoints and professional interests and is used in many ways such as in media contacts, in drafting legislation and testifying before congressional or legislative groups, and for communication with the public. A position paper is described as a statement of the association's stance on an issue that affects the nutritional status of the public; it is derived from pertinent facts and data and is germane to the ADA's mission, vision, philosophy, and values. Position papers are periodically updated or deleted and others added by the House of Delegates. The list of current position papers is shown in Appendix E and copies are available from the ADA headquarters office or at www.eatright.org.

AFFILIATED UNITS OF THE AMERICAN DIETETIC ASSOCIATION

State and District Associations

Each of the 50 states and Puerto Rico are affiliates of the ADA and are organized with state- and district-level associations. Membership in the ADA determines the membership in state affiliates. States generally charge no membership fees, but instead receive rebates from the ADA according to the number of members. A member of the ADA is automatically a member of a state affiliate.

The state organizations generally parallel the national organization. Each state elects its delegates to represent its members' interests in the HOD. District organizations are formed within a state and the number varies, determined by the state as well as how they fit into the state organization. The district and state groups provide educational and informational programs for the grassroots members. Most states have one or two meetings per year to conduct business and provide continuing education opportunities for the members. Delegates from the state affiliates take state and/or member issues to the HOD for all members to have input as state issues often lead to national issues.

American Dietetic Association Foundation

The American Dietetic Association Foundation is a nonprofit arm of the association that solicits and receives monies to benefit the association, with a large proportion of the monies going to provide scholarships for both undergraduate and graduate students and for member research projects. The foundation fosters alignment with corporate sponsors as well as conducts member campaigns for fundraising.

The foundation provides services for both members and the public. More than 900 students have been awarded scholarships in the last 5 years, totaling nearly $1.4 million. The Evidence Analysis Library, a resource offered through the foundation, is a member-accessible online reference library housing relevant nutritional research on important dietetic practice questions. The service is also available to others through a subscription service.[11]

Washington Office

Since 1986, the association has staffed an office in Washington, D.C., in order to have a presence in the capital and to further the legislative efforts of the profession. This proximity allows the association to keep informed of legislative issues as they are being considered and as they occur. Although legislative and lobbying efforts required a tax status change for the association when first initiated, the benefits accrue directly to individual members and indirectly to consumers and the public.

The staff of the Washington office and ADA members work with legislators and government agencies to introduce and promote bills that further the interests of the profession and its members. An example of successful legislation was the 2007 passage of the Medicare Medical Nutrition Therapy bill that resulted from a sustained effort on the part of the ADA staff working closely with legislators. As a result of the successful passage of this bill, dietitians could be reimbursed for dietetic services provided to persons with diabetes and/or kidney disease.

A yearly public policy workshop provides members with training opportunities in legislation and key issues to discuss with their congressional delegates.

SUMMARY

The ADA is the professional organization serving and promoting the interests of its members. The programs and initiatives administered by the association are for the benefits of the members and the public. The ADA is governed by elected and appointed volunteer members of boards, commissions, and committees, all of whom perform specific functions according to the bylaws of the ADA. Important as the functions are that the ADA provides for members, the association is recognized as the authoritative voice to the public for guidance regarding food and nutrition issues.

The active promotion of policy that enhances the health and well-being of all individuals is accomplished through activities by members and by the Washington legislative office.

DEFINITIONS

Bylaws. Authoritative rules and regulations governing an association or group.

Chief Executive Officer. A person employed by an association to direct and manage personnel, fiscal affairs, and programs of the association.

Governance. Activities involved in conducting the affairs of an organization.

Strategic Plan. Operational plans and goals that shape the overall activities and functions of an organization.

REFERENCES

1. Fitz, P. "The American Dietetic Association." *J Am Diet Assoc* 97(1997): 667–669.
2. ADA's Strategic Plan Effective June 2008. www.eatright.org (Accessed November 8, 2008).
3. See note 2.
4. Switt, J.T. "The American Dietetic Association's New Look." *J Am Diet Assoc* 108(2008): 932–933.
5. Lipscomb, R. "2008 ADA Member Benefits Update." *J Am Diet Assoc* 108(2008): 602–606.
6. Cassell, J. *Carry the Flame: The History of the American Dietetic Association.* The American Dietetic Association: Chicago; 1990.
7. Baldyga, W.W. "Results from the 1981 Census of the American Dietetic Association." *J Am Diet Assoc* 83(1983): 343–348.
8. Rogers, D. "Report on the ADA 2002 Dietetics Compensation and Benefits Survey." *J Am Diet Assoc* 103(2003): 243–255.
9. Rogers, D. "Compensation and Benefits Survey 2007: Above-Average Pay Gains Seen for Registered Dietitians." *J Am Diet Assoc* 108(2008): 416–427.
10. American Dietetic Association. Compensation and Benefits Survey of the Dietetics Profession 2009. www.eatright.org. Accessed October 25, 2009.
11. ADA. www.eatright.org (Accessed March 9, 2009).

Part II

Education and Professional Development

CHAPTER 3

Educational Preparation in Dietetics

"As a profession, the one thing that we can predict is that the greatest change in our practice will be the change in knowledge and how we integrate new science into our daily practice."[1]

OUTLINE

- Introduction
- Undergraduate Education
- Program Requirements
- Dietetics Education Requirements
  - Foundation Knowledge and Competencies
- Dietetics Education Programs
  - Didactic Program in Dietetics (DPD)
  - Coordinated Program in Dietetics (CP)
  - Dietetic Technician Program (DT)
- Trends in Dietetics Education
- Supervised Practice in Dietetics: Dietetic Internship
- Advanced-Level Education
  - Types of Programs
  - Benefits of Advanced Study
  - The Graduate Program Experience
  - Research Experience
- Summary

INTRODUCTION

Education is the key to dietetic practice and to the future of the profession. As with all professions, a specialized body of knowledge is required of individuals who practice in any area of dietetics. Because of the importance of education to the profession, the early leaders in dietetics set standards for education. The standards have been revised at intervals as the practice evolved and the needs of those being served changed.

UNDERGRADUATE EDUCATION

The educational preparation of dietitians begins in the undergraduate degree program. Study for the baccalaureate degree is based in the biological, physical, and social sciences and includes both a theoretical and applied course of study. The college or university offering a degree program plans a curriculum that meets both the educational standards of the American Dietetic Association and the university requirements, including courses for general education. A baccalaureate degree from an accredited college or university, combined with supervised practice integrated into the degree program, or an internship following the degree are necessary to complete all education requirements. A program that offers the practical experience component concurrent with the degree is termed a Coordinated Program (CP). A curriculum that meets the ADA education standards is referred to as a Didactic Program in Dietetics (DPD). The dietetic technician (DT) similarly follows a course of study in a 2-year college or institute that includes or is followed by supervised practice experience.

PROGRAM REQUIREMENTS

The Commission on Accreditation for Dietetics Education (CADE) sets the standards by which dietitians are educated. The standards have been issued in various forms since 1924 and have undergone many changes in concept and format.[2] For instance, early emphasis was on the specific courses a student was required to take during a degree program. Now, the standards are based on the outcomes expected from the education experience, and education program directors translate the expected outcomes into courses and course content.[3] CADE further specifies how a degree program is to be structured, including the goals and philosophy of the program, the students, the curriculum, the program resources, and the evaluation of the program.

Three CADE program standards are specified as follows:[4]

Standard One: program planning and outcomes assessment. The dietetics education program has clearly defined a mission, goals, program outcomes, and assessment measures, and implements a systematic, continuous process to assess outcomes, evaluate goal achievement, and improve program effectiveness.

Standard Two: Curriculum and student learning outcomes. The dietetics education program has a planned curriculum that provides for achievement of student learning outcomes and expected competence of the graduate.

Standard Three: Program management. Management of the dietetics education program and availability of program resources are evident in defined processes and procedures and demonstrate accountability to students and the public.

CADE evaluates each educational program through a site visit based on an extensive self-study prepared by the program director and staff. The purpose of the site visit by Registered Dietitians designated by the ADA is to assist the program in continual assessment that ensures qualified, competent program graduates. A program may be accredited for a period of 1 to 10 years. Periodic reports are submitted by the program director to the ADA indicating that a program continues to provide education that meets all standards.

A list of all accredited programs is available from a college or university department or from the ADA (www.eatright.org). The dietetics major is offered in at least one university in each state and in Hawaii and Puerto Rico.

DIETETICS EDUCATION REQUIREMENTS

The route to becoming a Registered Dietitian is based on the study of a wide variety of topics focusing on food, nutrition, and management. These areas are supported by the sciences: biological, physiological, behavioral, social, and communication. A combination of academic preparation including a baccalaureate degree and a supervised practice component completes the preparation for entry-level practice.

Foundation Knowledge and Competencies

The current educational standards were issued in 2008 after an extensive review and validation of the principles and criteria used, with input from faculty, administrators, students, practitioners, and employers.[5] This resulted in the development by CADE of a set of "Foundation Knowledge and Competencies" that are followed by programs in planning the curriculum. The learning outcomes from the use of these standards are outlined under five areas:

1. The scientific and evidence base of practice: Integration of scientific information and research into practice.
2. Professional practice expectations: Beliefs, values, attitudes, and behaviors for the professional dietitian level of practice.
3. Clinical and customer services: Development and delivery of information, products, and services to individuals, groups, and populations.
4. Practice management and use of resources: Strategic application of principles of management and systems in the provision of services to individuals and organizations.
5. Support knowledge: Knowledge underlying the requirements.

DIETETICS EDUCATION PROGRAMS

Didactic Program in Dietetics (DPD)

The didactic, or classwork, portion of the dietetics educational requirements is completed during the degree program (either undergraduate or graduate). Following degree conferral, the student completes a supervised practice program or internship. The traditional DPD is a 4-year undergraduate bachelor of science degree. Many of the courses required in the DPD combine classroom and laboratory work, especially courses in food production, clinical nutrition, and science courses such as chemistry and microbiology. During the later part of the program, usually the senior year, the student applies to one or more dietetic internships through a computerized matching program. Notification is given in April or November about a "match" or acceptance to the student's program of choice.

This program is followed by the dietetic internship, after which the student may take the registration exam.

Coordinated Program in Dietetics (CP)

In the CP, the didactic portion of a program and supervised practice are completed during the course of study towards the degree, either undergraduate or graduate. The student graduating from this program is thus prepared for entry-level practice upon completion of the degree. In most universities, students enter the CP for their junior and senior years. The program is sometimes referred to as "two by two," meaning the first 2 years are general study and may be at a community or junior college and the last 2 include the integrated courses leading to the degree. Some programs may be longer than the traditional 4 years depending on the specific program requirements.

A university designates the criteria for admission to the CP. The selection criteria commonly include grade point average, writing skill, work experience, letters of recommendation, and sometimes, an interview. A minimum of 1200 clock hours of supervised practice is required in the CP. The CP is intense in terms of time requirements and experiences but can reduce the time needed to prepare for practice. On completion of the degree, the student is eligible to take the registration examination.

Dietetic Technician Program (DT)

The DT program is similar to the coordinated program in that both didactic knowledge and skills and supervised practice (a minimum of 450 clock hours) are required in the program. The requirements are specified and programs are accredited by CADE. Graduates of the program are eligible to take the registration examination for DTs and for entry-level practice. Many of these programs are offered in 2-year colleges or in technical schools.

TRENDS IN DIETETICS EDUCATION

The education of the dietitian must be focused on the present and future practice roles the professionals are expected to fulfill. The traditional roles continue to expand as environmental, demographic, business, and health trends create new opportunities for practice.

In 2006, the ADA House of Delegates conducted an environmental scan to identify, prioritize, and evaluate trends affecting the profession of dietetics.[6] Members were asked to help identify the trends that challenge and perhaps even change the direction of the profession. The 11 themes identified in the study are the following:

1. Aging
2. The high obesity rate
3. A fast-food, eat-and-run society
4. The global explosion in communications
5. Growth of diversity among the U.S. population
6. A maturing industrialized food system
7. Economic gaps between the "haves" and "have-nots"
8. Environmental issues
9. Policy focus on health and wellness
10. Alternative health care
11. Science and technology burgeoning potential

Summaries of the potential implications are included in the study report.

These trends have a number of implications for the education of the dietitian because practice changes as societal factors influence health care in various ways. Continuing education is also a "must" for the practicing professional in order to keep abreast of new developments, anticipated change, and for planning ahead.

In 2003, a task force on dietetics education was appointed by the House of Delegates.[7] The task force was to begin creation of a new plan for the future of education and credentialing for RDs and DTRs and for the education of advanced-level dietetics professionals. In 2006, the group submitted seven recommendations that were discussed by the HOD. A Phase 2 "Future Practice and Education" task force was then assigned to continue the planning. Their final report was submitted in 2008.[8] The recommendations concerned DTR education and practice, innovative quality education models for entry-level RD programs, specialty practice, future advanced practice, and resource allocation. One recommendation that the HOD appoint a council on Future Practice and Education has been implemented. This council will work in collaboration with CDR and CADE to project the future practice needs for the profession of dietetics. Each of these organizational units (future practice credentialing, and accreditations) represent the three critical segments necessary for producing new practitioners, as well as assisting experienced practitioners to move up the career ladder. Further discussion and action is anticipated.

SUPERVISED PRACTICE IN DIETETICS: DIETETIC INTERNSHIP

Preprofessional or supervised practice is an essential step toward becoming an RD or a DTR. For the DPD student the dietetic internship follows the degree. Supervised practice takes place in the work setting where students learn to apply their knowledge and skills under the direction of an RD preceptor. Successful completion of a supervised practice program establishes eligibility for an individual to write the registration examination and to apply for active membership in the ADA. Competency in dietetics practice is the goal of supervised practice. Competency is regarded as the ability to carry out tasks within certain expected standards or parameters.

Supervised practice programs are based on the standards of education and the performance requirements for entry-level practice. All supervised programs are provided through an accredited program and must offer a minimum of 1200 clock hours of experience for the dietitian and 450 clock hours for the dietetic technician. A current listing of all programs is available in *The Directory of Dietetics Programs* from the ADA.[9] The directory provides information about the length of the program, the number of students per class, estimated tuition, availability of financial aid, credit given toward an advanced degree, and the due date for the next accreditation survey.

All supervised practice programs follow the same standards, however, there is flexibility in how the programs meet the standards. Although CADE accredits programs, it does not mandate the kinds of experiences or the amount of time in each area of practice. Each program sets the curriculum and experiences that meet the goals of the program and the needs of the student.

Program experiences are structured around three key areas of activity in dietetics: clinical nutrition, food service management, and community dietetics. Programs that do not offer all the experiences in one institution will arrange with others in the community to provide them.

The dietetic internship, the CP, and the DT programs are the three types of supervised programs. The following questions are often asked when students apply to supervised practice programs:

What do students need to know before applying? Students should know that a period of supervised experience is required to establish eligibility to become an RD or DT and that acceptance into a program is competitive. Further, the application process should begin early in the senior year in order to assemble all required materials by graduation and, if required by the program or desired by the student, to visit the program. Students applying for a dietetic internship usually will be required to participate in national computer matching, and this information may be obtained from the program director or from the ADA office.

What are the characteristics of successful applicants? Generally, those applicants with a grade point average of 3.0 or above in food, nutrition, and management courses and better than average grades in biological and physical science courses will be considered first. Approximately 1 year of work experience or dietetics-related volunteer or paid experience will increase the chances of being accepted.

What else is important to know? In addition to good grades and having work experience, applicants are encouraged to investigate programs early to identify the specific admission criteria and to apply to one or more programs. Successful applicants often apply to as many as three programs. If the program offers graduate credit during the supervised experience, the student will also need to apply to graduate school and complete the Graduate Record Exam (GRE). In addition, applicants are encouraged to be flexible and be willing to relocate if necessary.

ADVANCED-LEVEL EDUCATION

Advanced-level education may be described as continuing or postprofessional education, or graduate education. More baccalaureate students are pursuing a graduate degree; more employers are requiring an advanced degree or training; and more disciplines are becoming specialized, thus requiring advanced-level education. Graduate education is formal study beyond a baccalaureate degree that leads to an advanced degree, usually the master's or doctoral degree. Graduate study involves concentrated study in a specific academic area. Some universities offer graduate study concurrently with the dietetic internship.

Among the important purposes of advanced education are opportunities for individuals to explore new ideas, and to gain the higher level of knowledge and understanding required to recognize and fully discharge personal, social, and professional responsibilities.[10] Practical benefits also accrue, including the possibility of career advancement and financial gains.

Types of Programs

The Master of Science (MS) degree usually requires 1 to 2 years of full-time study and may be longer depending on the major area of study, the research undertaken, and whether the student is employed while working toward the degree. In some universities, the MS is offered with the option of a thesis or a creative component instead of the thesis, entailing either extra course work or a project.

The doctor of philosophy (PhD) degree requires at least 3 to 5 years of full-time study. The PhD or the EdD (Doctor of Education) may be offered. Original research is required for either degree, the type depending on the field of study. The doctoral degree is considered the "terminal degree," although it may be followed by postdoctoral academic work.

A comparison of dietetics education requirements with those of 16 other health professions was reported by Skipper and Lewis.[11] The findings show that dietetics education is of shorter duration than for most of the other professions compared. This disparity may highlight the need for the profession to encourage the development of advanced-study programs that help practitioners who are in or are aspiring to advanced-level positions.

Benefits of Advanced Study

Although an advanced degree is not required to take the registration examination in dietetics, there are valid reasons for dietitians to pursue advanced study. In the 2009 Dietetics Compensation and Benefits Survey, it was reported that 50 percent of RDs hold an advanced degree. Among DTRs, 28 percent hold a bachelor's degree or higher.[12]

The benefits of an advanced degree include the development of intellectual skills, including the ability to master complex information; to problem solve; and to explore new ideas. Career benefits include the development of advanced practice skills, the in-depth exploration of subjects in one's area of practice, and the acquisition of new perspectives.[13] Dietitians often pursue graduate study for career advancement or preparation for a career change. Dietitians who are prepared to perform in multi-skilled or cross-trained positions will usually rely on graduate education to increase both knowledge and practice skills. The types of positions dietitians assume as they progress up the career ladder are usually those with increasing responsibility and autonomy, and they require managerial and leadership skills. In addition, competition for jobs may increase the demand for an advanced degree. New and expanding career options, and the job market in general, affect demand and availability of persons prepared to enter the new job markets and, in turn, influence dietitians in their education choices. Graduate education provides an opportunity to develop expertise that allows dietitians to assume leadership roles.

The financial advantages of an advanced degree for RDs are demonstrated in Table 3-1. Attaining an advanced degree increases the yearly wages of Registered Dietitians by $6000 (MS) and $29,000 (PhD). State licensure and specialty certification also affect salaries, and are often equated with advanced study. Dietitians working in practice areas that often require an advanced degree, such as food and nutrition management, consultation and business, and education and research, earn the highest salaries (Table 2-2).

For DTRs, the median wage was $36,400 in 1997 and $40,000 in 2009.[14] Factors affecting these salaries are the same as for the RD: education, experience, responsibility, and location. The DTRs in food and nutrition management or consultation and business earn the highest salaries.

Table 3-1. Median Yearly Income of Registered Dietitians by Education Level

	2007[1]	2009[2]
All RDs	$53,000	$57,000
Doctoral degree	78,000	83,000
Master's degree	56,000	60,000
Bachelor's degree	50,000	54,000

Sources: 1. Rogers, D. "Compensation and Benefits Survey 2007: Above Average Pay Gains Seen for Registered Dietitians." *J Am Diet Assoc* 108(2008): 416–427.

2. American Dietetic Association. Compensation and Benefits Survey of the Dietetics Profession 2009. www.eatright.org. Accessed October 20, 2009.

A further justification for the RD to pursue graduate study is for continuing education credit to maintain registration status. State licensure regulations often mandate an advanced degree and continuing education as well.

Active membership in the ADA is available to an individual holding a master's or doctoral degree in one of the following areas: dietetics, food and nutrition, food science, or food service systems management. The degree must be from a regionally accredited college or university.

Gaining research skills and understanding research articles and reports is a further benefit of graduate study. All dietitians apply research in their practice and need to demonstrate the ability to interpret current research and basic statistics. However, designing and participating in more formal research usually occur at the graduate level.

The Graduate Program Experience

Information about graduate programs offering degrees in dietetics or closely related subject areas is available in the ADA Directory of Programs or from universities. Prospective students will find it helpful to talk with faculty and to request college catalogs and departmental information before applying. No two programs are alike, and the best fit between the student and a program will be important once the student is admitted. Universities that give students an active role in departmental activities and who give individual time and attention in a mentoring and supportive atmosphere will greatly enhance the graduate experience. The faculty, departmental research, and the availability of financial aid through graduate assistantships should also be explored. Assistantships not only provide financial aid but give the student teaching, research, and/or administrative experience according to assignments.

Research Experience

The selection of a research study by the student with an advisor is based on the area of interest, the need as determined by a literature search, and the feasibility (cost, time involvement, availability of equipment and/or subjects). Ongoing departmental research by faculty can provide a way for the student to assume a part of the research for his or her thesis.

The process of investigating a problem, reviewing the literature to support the need for the study, planning and implementing the study, collecting and analyzing data, and writing a clear and well-developed document that is accepted by a graduate faculty committee is a significant effort. The research experience requires initiative, critical thinking, problem-solving, and ethics. These are aspects of professional functions that are vital to success in life, as well as a career. The successful completion of a research study often launches a student into publishing the results and into further research, thus making an important contribution to scholarship.

SUMMARY

Dietetics education has evolved over time but has always been based on preparing the student for professional practice. The ADA designates the educational standards that are followed by all dietetics programs, thus ensuring competent practitioners. With a background of academic knowledge and practical skills, dietitians and dietetic technicians are prepared for a wide variety of careers as described in other chapters in this book.

Almost half of practicing dietitians today hold or are working toward a graduate degree. There are benefits in doing so, among them the attainment of research competence, continuing education for personal and professional growth, and career enhancement. If the trend continues, ever-larger numbers of dietitians will seek an advanced degree and will thereby bring expertise to bear on practical problems in food, nutrition, and health. The outcome will be a healthy and informed public and heightened recognition of the dietitian as the expert in food and nutrition.

DEFINITIONS

Accreditation. The process whereby a private nongovernmental agency or association grants public recognition to an institution or an individual that meets necessary qualifications and periodic evaluations.

Coordinated Program. A degree program combining didactic and experiential learning.

Didactic Instruction. Knowledge acquired through classroom instruction.

Preceptor. A person who guides, mentors, and evaluates a student during the supervised practice experience.

Supervised Practice. Learning experiences associated with activities in selected situations that enable the student to apply knowledge, develop and retain skills, and develop professionally.

REFERENCES

1. Parks, S.C., M.R. Schiller, and J. Bryk. "President's Page: Investment in Our Future—The Role of Science and Scholarship in Developing Knowledge for Dietetics Practice." *J Am Diet Assoc* 94(1994): 1159–1161.
2. Wenberg, K., B.E. Mitchell, and M.M. Pfeiffer. "Dietetics Education: Past, Present, and Future." In *Proceedings of Future Search Conference Challenging the Future of Dietetics Education and Credentialing—Dialogue, Discovery, and Directions.* The American Dietetic Association and Commission on Registration: Chicago; 1994, pp. 3–12.
3. Commission on Accreditation for Dietetics Education. "Eligibility Requirements and Accreditation Standards for Programs in Dietetics." www.eatright.org (Accessed November 3, 2008).
4. Ibid.
5. Ibid.
6. Jarratt, J. and J.B. Mahaffie. "The Profession of Dietetics at a Critical Juncture: A Report on the 2006 Environmental Scan for the American Dietetic Association." *J Am Diet Assoc* 107, no. 7(2007): 39–57.
7. Task Force Report and Recommendations. "Dietetics Education Task Force." www.eatright.org (Accessed April 5, 2005). House of Delegates. American Dietetic Association; March 21, 2005.
8. Final Report of the Phase 2 Future Practice and Education Task Force. Education Task Force, House of Delegates, American Dietetic Association July 15, 2008. www.eatright.org (Accessed July 20, 2008).
9. Directory of Dietetics Education Programs by State-Media. www.eatright.org (Accessed March 10, 2009).
10. Brooks, P. "Point of View. Graduate Learning as Apprenticeship." Abstract. *Chronicle of Higher Education* XLIII(1996): A52.
11. Skipper, A. and N.M. Lewis. "A Look at the Educational Preparation of the Health-Diagnosing and Treating Professions: Do Dietitians Measure Up?" *J Am Diet Assoc* 105(2005): 420–427.
12. American Dietetic Association. Compensation and Benefits Survey of the Dietetic Profession 2009. www.eatright.org. Accessed October 20, 2009.
13. Gaffney, N.A. *Graduate School and You: A Guide for Prospective Graduate Students,* 4th ed. Washington, D.C.: Council on Graduate Schools; 1996.
14. American Dietetic Association. Compensation and Benefits Survey of the Dietetic Profession 2009. www.eatright.org. Accessed October 20, 2009.

CHAPTER 4

Credentialing of Dietetic Practitioners

"Experts at curing diseases are inferior to specialists who warn against disease. Experts in the use of medicines are inferior to those who recommend proper diet."[1]

OUTLINE

- Introduction
- Development of Credentialing
- Commission on Dietetic Registration (CDR)
  - Registered Dietitian (RD)
  - Dietetic Technician, Registered (DTR)
  - New DTR Registration Eligibility Pathway
  - Specialist Certification
  - Certificates of Training
  - Recertification of the RD and DTR
  - Recertification of Specialists
  - Appropriate Use of Credentials
- Legal Regulation of Dietitians and Nutritionists
- Summary

INTRODUCTION

The term dietitian was one that evolved over time. Early practitioners were called dietologists, dietists, and dietotherapists.[2] Before the American Dietetic Association (ADA) was formed, a dietitian was described as "a

51

person who specializes in the knowledge of food and can meet the demands of the medical profession for diet therapy."[2] This adequately described the professional for many decades.

The developing science of food and nutrition formed the basis for the organization of a group of practicing professionals. One of the earliest concerns of this group was the overwhelming amount of food faddism and fallacies found among the general public and even other professionals. It was difficult, if not impossible, for the public to determine who was a credible source of information and to separate fact from fiction between the many medical and health claims for specific foods and procedures.

This early concern for protection of the public by disseminating the knowledge of dietitians has continued to the present time. Not only did it lead to the national organization of dietitians that could promote the professionals as having expertise in "diet-therapy, teaching, social welfare, and administration,"[3] but it served as the impetus to begin thinking about credentialing of practitioners.

A concern raised at the second annual meeting of the ADA in 1918 was the "need to distinguish between dietitians with a college degree and special training in some scientific work and the ones with lesser training."[4]

This was perhaps the first formal reference to dietetic credentialing. The 1926 president of the association, Florence Smith, urged that the group establish professional standards for dietitians and that state or national registration could be the answer. In 1929, a study of national registration was initiated and the following definition of a dietitian was adopted: "Any person who is qualified for membership in The American Dietetic Association is by virtue of uniform basic training and required experience, entitled to be designated as a dietitian."[5] In the 1950s the association appointed a committee to formally study state licensing of dietitians. The issue of specialties in practice also surfaced with the suggestion that membership should be expanded to include others who were well qualified in the many specialties embraced within the definition of dietetics.[6] However, it was in the late 1990s that education and membership requirements were differentiated to accommodate practitioners with similar basic preparation but in specialized areas of practice.

The differences between a generalist and a specialist surfaced and were thoroughly debated. A generalist was defined as a dietitian who could perform in all areas of practice, such as a single dietitian in a small hospital, or one who could move from one practice area to another. A specialist was a dietitian wanting to restrict his or her practice in one area, such as clinical or food service.

The generalist role was advanced by the following themes:

1. All dietitians are the same.
2. Dietitians can move from one area of practice to another (food service to public health, for example) without additional training.
3. Greater external recognition of the term dietitian was established.

By contrast, the specialized role was driven by the following themes:

1. The explosion of knowledge and technology required each dietitian to know more and more about less and less.
2. There was a need to differentiate among dietitians with varying skills and knowledge, advanced education, and experience gained on the job.
3. Part-time employment opportunities emerged.
4. New, innovative practice areas developed, such as school food service, nursing home consultation, enteral and parenteral nutrition techniques, and nutrition support.

DEVELOPMENT OF CREDENTIALING

In the 1960s a committee was established to study licensure, registration, and certification. Registration was the credentialing process chosen at that time by the ADA House of Delegates and the ADA membership. An amendment to the constitution was approved for the "Final Revised Proposal for Professional Registration" in 1969. A committee, later to become known as the Commission on Dietetic Registration (CDR), then began the implementation of a certification process for members. The title for those ADA members who chose to become certified was Registered Dietitian (RD). A detailed account of the implementation and a review of the first 5 years of professional registration were published in the *Journal of the American Dietetic Association* in 1974.[7]

The professional registration system adopted by the association differed significantly from other health professional certification systems at that time in that candidates had to pass a national examination, and Registered Dietitians (RDs) had to document evidence of continuing education in each 5-year period to renew registration. Thus registration was designed as a voluntary process to ensure competency of dietitians through the qualifications required to take the registration examination, passing the examination, and formal continuing education. All of this was evidence of the concern of the profession for the health, safety, and welfare of the public by encouraging high standards of performance by dietetic practitioners as stated in the amendment to the constitution.[8]

Ninety percent of the membership was registered by the end of the 1970s, with the majority "grandfathered" in during the period before establishment of the examination. Credentialing of the dietetic technician and various dietetic specialists followed with qualifications developed by the Commission on Dietetic Registration.

COMMISSION ON DIETETIC REGISTRATION (CDR)

The Commission on Dietetic Registration (CDR) is the agency responsible for maintaining the registration process for the ADA. This group develops the examination for registration and sets the standards for certification, recertification, and the code of ethics and issues credentials to individuals who meet these standards.[9] Their mission statement is:

"Protecting the nutritional health and welfare of the public through dietetics certification."

Registered Dietitian (RD)

The examination to become an RD is administered online (prior to this advancement it was offered in written form at designated sites twice a year) and is available whenever an applicant chooses. The examination is also available in other countries with which the ADA has reciprocity. The process by which the 75 clock hours of continuing education are accumulated is also determined by the CDR, which specifies the educational activities that qualify for recertification as an RD.

The eligibility requirements for dietitians to take the examination for RD are the following:[10]

1. Education. Minimum of a baccalaureate degree from an accredited college or university and completion of the current Standards of Education as approved by the Commission on Accreditation for Dietetics Education (CADE) of the ADA. Additional information and updates can be found at www.eatright.org and click on Commission on Dietetic Registration or Commission on Accreditation for Dietetics Education.

2. Supervised practice. To be fulfilled in an accredited dietetic internship or accredited coordinated program. The Web site above will also provide current information as to the type and length of supervised practice required.

Dietetic Technician, Registered (DTR)

The Dietetic Technician, Registered is a critical member of the dietetics team and becomes even more important as the practice of dietetics in every area becomes more complicated and time consuming. Dietetic technicians are trained in food and nutrition and are an integral part of health care, food service, and other dietetics and healthcare teams. In small, rural hospitals the DTR is sometimes the only trained dietetics practitioner addressing all aspects of care available full-time. In this situation, the DTR works under the supervision of an RD via established protocols to implement the nutrition care process based on state regulations. At present, only Maine has state licensure procedures for the dietetic technician. "The Scope of Dietetic Practice Framework" guidelines for licensure document addresses supervision, entry-level, and advanced practice for DTRs.[11]

The role of the dietetic technician must be recognized, strengthened, and supported. An increase in the number of DTRs is vital to sustain expansion of practice areas for dietitians and achieve the future vision for the profession.

The small number of DTRs and dietetic technician educational programs place this segment of our profession at risk for continued existence. Steps must be taken to ensure a sufficient number of DTRs to meet demand and achieve the future vision of the dietetics team who need DTRs as viable team members to succeed.

In addition a realistic and workable career ladder within the dietetics profession must be created and implemented as quickly as possible. The opportunity for advancement, moving from dietetic technician to Registered Dietitian to advanced practitioner, must become a reality. A functional career ladder strengthens the dietetics profession as we seek to enhance the recognition, authority, autonomy, prestige, income, and satisfaction of dietetics team members and their customers.

It is well known that DTRs work in non-traditional or emerging areas of practice with more diverse possibilities for the future. After years of practice DTRs also may work with RDs in advanced-level practice areas such as renal dietetics. The use of the "Standards of Practice" and "Standards of Professional Performance for Dietetic Technicians, Registered" partially addresses this issue of advanced practice for DTRs.[12] The DTR works under the direction of the RD in the provision of clinical nutrition services or medical nutrition therapy. The DTR practices in food service management, community programs, and in evolving settings and organizational structures. Depending on the complexity of the organization, the DTR may or may not work under the supervision of the RD.

The opportunities for employment keep expanding for the DTR, especially in areas where supply of RDs cannot meet the demand. More and more positions, especially in the healthcare arena, are requiring that an individual be credentialed as a DTR in order to practice in the facilities. Some current unique opportunities are:

- Supervising food safety and sanitation in a variety of public and private venues
- Assisting individuals and groups in wellness and fitness centers to know how food relates to fitness
- Managing and directing food service employees in assisted living and retirement centers
- Assisting the RD in collecting data from patients or participants in a research study (in hospitals, clinics, and community research centers)

The "2008 Final Report of the Phase 2 Future Practice and Education Task Force" provides much detail of innovative educational experiences and unique roles and employment for DTRs both now and in the future.[13]

The DTR of today will extend the scope of practice for the RD in the future and will allow the RDs to delegate responsibilities enabling them to practice at specialty and advanced levels. However, for this to happen the RD must understand the role and appropriate responsibilities of the DTR, which in many instances will increase visibility and credibility of the dietetic professional team and will benefit clients, facilities, the RD, and the profession of dietetics. Last but not least, the dietetics profession and the ADA must promote the value of DTR educational programs and the dietetic technician as a creditable member of the team for practice in tomorrow's world.

New DTR Registration Eligibility Pathway

For the past several years the CDR and others have noted the decline of the number of DTRs. This decline has been complicated by the lack of educational programs for DTRs in many states, in other words many employers have been unable to hire DTRs, which has increased the unavailability of DTRs in many parts of the United States. The CDR has supported the role of the dietetic technician and believes that a new pathway will address both of these issues. This decision is consistent with the CDR's public protection mission in that it provides a credential for the numerous non-credentialed DPD graduates currently employed in dietetic technician positions. Once credentialed as a DTR, these individuals will be required to comply with the CDR recertification requirements and the "Code of Ethics for the Profession of Dietetics and the Standards of Practice."[14] The CDR also believes that this alternative registration eligibility option will provide a dietetics career ladder, increase the availability and visibility of DTRs throughout the country, and ultimately enhance the value of the DTR credential.

Therefore, at its April 2009 meeting the CDR established a new registration eligibility pathway for dietetic technicians. Effective June 1, 2009, individuals who have completed both a baccalaureate degree and a Didactic Program in Dietetics (DPD) will be able to take the registration examination for dietetic technicians without meeting additional academic or supervised practice requirements. This decision also provides for the numerous non-credentialed DPD graduates currently employed in dietetic technician positions to become credentialed. Once credentialed, these individuals will be required to comply with CDR recertification requirements and the "Code of Ethics for the Profession of Dietetics and the Standards of Practice." CDR also believes that this alternative registration eligibility option will increase the availability and visibility of DTRs throughout the country ultimately enhancing the value of the DTR credential.

Effective June 1, 2009, the three pathways to establish eligibility to take the registration examination for dietetic technicians are:

1. Original Pathway I. Completion of an associate's degree granted by a U.S. regionally accredited college or university with the (CADE) Accredited Dietetic Technician Program.
2. Original Pathway II. Completion of a baccalaureate degree granted by a U.S. regionally accredited college or university, or foreign equivalent, completion of a CADE Didactic Program in Dietetics (DPD), and completion of a CADE-accredited dietetic technician supervised practice.
3. New Pathway. Completion of a baccalaureate degree granted by a U.S. regionally accredited college or university, or foreign equivalent, and completion of a CADE Didactic Program in Dietetics (DPD) or Coordinated Program in Dietetics (CP).

For security reasons, all candidates must be processed through the Credential Registration and Maintenance System (CRMS) for eligibility to take the examination issued by their DPD Program Director. All candidates must complete an electronic application in PDF writeable format, available on CDR's Web site at: http://www.cdrnet.org/pdfs/DTRPathway3.pdf.

The following are additional ADA Web sites of importance to dietetic technicians:

DTRE Mis-Use:
  http://www.cdrnet.org/PDFs/DTRE%20%20Mis-Use%20%20
  -%20%20Updated%204-09.pdf
Examination Candidate Information and Study Resources
Computer-Based Testing FAQ:
  http://www.cdrnet.org/certifications/rddtr/cbtfaq.htm
Study Guide for the Registration Examination for Dietetic Technicians, 5th edition:
  http://www.eatright.org/cps/rde/xchg/ada/hs.xsl/shop_9603_ENU_
  HTML.htm
"Check It Out—Becoming a Dietetic Technician Registered":
  http://www.eatright.org/ada/files/DTR_Check_it_Out(1).PDF

Specialist Certification

In 1986, the concept of specialized practice in dietetics was approved by the House of Delegates. The ADA defined a specialty as an advanced level of practice that responds to a defined area of need and requires demonstrated competency exceeding that for entry-level practice. Specialty areas must have a substantial and verifiable knowledge base, an identified dimension of advanced practice, and a reasonably sized pool of practitioners. Three areas of practice were selected for initial certification: pediatric nutrition, renal nutrition, and metabolic nutrition care.[15] The first specialty areas were chartered in 1994. The metabolic nutrition care specialty was later discontinued.[16] Currently specialists are certified in the following areas:

> Board Certified Specialist in Gerontological Nutrition (CSG)
> Board Certified Specialist in Sports Dietetics (CSSD)
> Board Certified Specialist in Pediatric Nutrition (CSP)
> Board Certified Specialist in Renal Nutrition (CSR)
> Board Certified Specialist in Oncology Nutrition (CSO)

An additional area of recognition was developed in 1993 for those practicing at advanced levels in any area of dietetics.[16] The "Fellow of the American Dietetic Association" was available until 2003 for those having an advanced degree, 8 years of practice, plus other documented professional achievements.[17] This recognition was discontinued because of limited participation of members of the association.[18]

Certificates of Training

Currently the CDR offers Certificates of Training in two areas. Responding to the epidemic of obesity and the need for Registered Dietitians to become more involved in the efforts to prevent and treat obesity CDR provides workshops across the United States resulting in certificates in Childhood and Adolescent Weight Management and in Adult Weight Management. The certificate programs are designed to develop practitioners of comprehensive weight management care for adults, children, and adolescents. The certificates are available for ADA members, RDs, and DTRs. Training for the certificates includes:

- State-of-the-art information and skills shared by leading practitioners
- Hands-on experience with cases and exercises

- Reference and other resource materials
- Twenty-nine hours of continuing professional education units

This training and subsequent certificates have become very useful and popular with dietetic professionals returning to the workplace, working in private practice, and to Registered Dietitians in general. There is no reissue of the certificates, but certificants are encouraged to participate in retraining as needed. Additional information can be found at the CDR Web site (www.cdrnet.org).

Recertification of the RD and DTR

In 2001, the CDR implemented a new process for continued certification termed the Professional Development Portfolio (PDP).[19] To maintain registered status, Registered Dietitians (RD) and Dietetic Technicians, Registered (DTR) must participate in CDR's mandatory PDP recertification system and remit the annual registration maintenance fee. Using this plan, the individual RD and DTR assumes the responsibility for learning, professional development, and career direction. The PDP requires each practitioner to first engage in self-reflection, followed by assessment and goal setting. This process is followed by the development of a 5-year plan that reflects a critical analysis of goals and the steps to be taken to maintain professional competency.[19,20]

Continuing professional education (CPE) is essential for lifelong development to maintain and improve knowledge and skills for competent dietetics practice. RDs and DTRs must report continuing professional education units (CPEUs) using the PDP recertification system. To remain registered, an RD is required to pay yearly dues and engage in 75 clock hours of continuing education over a 5-year period. A DTR pays dues and must accrue 50 clock hours in a 5-year period.

Recertification of Specialists

The Specialty Board Certification is a practice credential (just as is RD and DTR) that represents to the public that the certificant possesses the knowledge, skills, and experience to function effectively as a specialist in that area. The nature of the knowledge and skills to practice at a specialty level is subject to change due to technological and scientific advances. Recertification testing helps to provide continuing assurance that the certified specialist has indeed maintained knowledge in his or her specialty area.

Therefore, at the end of the specialist's 5-year certification period, those who wish to recertify in the same specialty area must meet the following criteria:

- Currently a Registered Dietitian with CDR
- Successfully complete an eligibility application
- Submit an application fee
- Provide documentation of the required minimum number of specialty practice hours
- Successfully complete a specialty examination

Appropriate Use of Credentials

In 1989, the Commission on Dietetic Registration (CDR) issued a statement on the protection of the credentials RD and DTR.[19] CDR recognized that the credentials that it controls are most valuable to it and to the holders of those credentials because they are awarded only to individuals who have met the education and experiential requirements and have passed appropriate examinations. Practitioners may use these credentials only if they continue to meet CDR requirements, including payment of a registration maintenance fee and fulfillment of the continuing education hours required. As noted in the statement: "The most common usage is after the practitioner's name as a professional designation, e.g., Jane Doe, RD or John Smith, DTR." Other specific details of the joint policy statement of the CDR and the ADA Board of Directors are included in the reference.[21]

LEGAL REGULATION OF DIETITIANS AND NUTRITIONISTS

Forty-six states now have laws that regulate dietitians or nutritionists through licensure, statutory certification, or registration. Thirty-one or 67 percent of these states have included the protection of a scope of practice as well as protection of the name Registered Dietitian; one-half of these states protect the title of nutritionist as well; Nebraska protects the title of medical nutrition therapist, and one state (Maine) has licensure for dietetic technicians. State licensure and state certification are entirely separate and distinct from registration or certification by the Commission on Dietetic Registration.

The 46 states that regulate dietitians or nutritionists do so through licensure, statutory certification, or registration. For state regulation purposes, these terms are defined as the following:

- Licensing. Statutes include an explicitly defined scope of practice, and performance of the profession is illegal without first obtaining a license from the state.
- Statutory certification. Limits use of particular titles to persons meeting predetermined requirements, while persons not certified can still practice the occupation or profession.
- Registration. The least restrictive form of state regulation. As with certification, unregistered persons are permitted to practice the profession. Typically, exams are not given and enforcement of the registration requirement is minimal.

Dietetics practitioners are licensed by states to ensure that only qualified, trained professional provide nutrition services or advice to individuals requiring or seeking nutrition care or dietetics information. In states with licensure, only state-licensed dietetics professionals can provide nutrition counseling and other services, included in the "Scope of Practice," as a part of the licensure law. Non-licensed practitioners may be subject to prosecution for practicing without a license. States with certification laws limit the use of particular titles (e.g., dietitian or nutritionist) to persons meeting predetermined requirements; however, persons not certified can still practice, but cannot hold themselves out as dietitians or use the title in their practice. Consumers in these states who are seeking nutrition therapy assistance need to be more cautious and aware of the qualifications of the provider they choose.

As dietitians or dietetic technicians travel from state to state to practice dietetics it is important to contact a state regulatory agency to determine state licensure law provisions prior to practicing dietetics. State licensure agency contact information can usually be obtained by contacting the State Dietetic Association or CDR who maintains a current list of states with licensure or certification laws in place.

SUMMARY

Dietitians continue to desire recognition and differentiation among their peers that is visible and can be communicated to other professional practitioners. The credentialing program does this. The RD has become valued to the point that most individuals consider it synonymous with dietitian. The same is becoming true for the DTR. Many employers view both as mandatory credentials to practice in various employment settings. Credentials also have been used in international markets and jobs to describe individuals and job qualifications. For dietitians, dietetic technicians, and dietetic specialists this is a plus as the world moves toward a global practice and global economy.

Consumers will always demand credentials of some kind. As consumers recognize that the credentials of the ADA provide assurance that the practitioners are competent and can provide services they want, the demand will continue to rise. More significantly, these credentials will enhance the dietetics professionals' efforts to describe the diversity of their capabilities and to obtain a competitive advantage in the practice of dietetics in the United States and internationally.

DEFINITIONS

Certification. The process by which a nongovernmental agency or association grants recognition to an individual who has met certain predetermined qualifications specified by that agency or association (e.g., registration for dietitians and dietetic technicians administered by the CDR).

Credentialing. Formal recognition of professional or technical competence as by certification or licensure.

Licensure. Process by which a government agency grants permission to an individual to engage in a given occupation upon finding that the applicant has attained the minimal degree of competency necessary to ensure that the public health, safety, and welfare are reasonably well protected.

Practitioner. One who practices in a profession or occupation.

Registration. See Certification.

Scope of Practice. Extent of or dimensions of activities performed in an area of practice.

REFERENCES

1. Needham, J. *Clerks and Craftsmen in China and the West. Lectures and Addresses on the History of the Science and Technology.* University Press: Cambridge, MA; 1970, p. 95.

2. Cassell, J. *Carry the Flame: The History of the American Dietetic Association.* The American Dietetic Association: Chicago; 1990, p. 9

3. Ibid. p. 22

4. Ibid. p. 26

5. Ibid. p. 71

6. Perry, E. "Report of the Executive Board." *J Am Diet Assoc* 26(1950): 949–957.

7. Bogle, M.L. "Registration: The *Sine Qua Non* of a Competent Dietitian." *J Am Diet Assoc* 74(1974): 616–620.

8. ADA. "Constitution of the American Dietetic Association, as Amended." The American Dietetic Association: Chicago; 1971.

9. ADA. "Bylaws of American Dietetic Association." Revised March 10, 2002. www.eatright.org/member/governance/85_12428.cfm (Accessed March 1, 2004).

10. Keim, K.S., CA. Johnson, and G.E. Gates. "Learning Needs and Continuing Professional Education Activities of Professional Development Portfolio Participants." *J Am Diet Assoc* 101, no. 6(2001): 697–702.

11. O'Sullivan-Maillet, J., J. Skates, and E. Pritchett. "Scope of Dietetics Practice Framework." *J Am Diet Assoc* 105(2005): 634–640.

12. ADA. "American Dietetic Association Revised 2008 Standards of Practice for Registered Dietitians in Nutrition Care; Standards of Professional Performance for Registered Dietitians; Standards of Practice for Dietetic Technicians, Registered; and Standards of Professional Performance for Dietetic Technicians, Registered." *J Am Diet Assoc* 108(2008): 1535–1542.

13. ADA. "Final Report of the Phase 2 Future Practice and Education Task Force." The American Dietetic Association: Chicago; 2008, pp. 2–72

14. ADA. "Commission on Dietetic Registration Code of Ethics for the Profession of Dietetics and Process for Consideration of Ethics Issues." *J Am Diet Assoc* 109(2009): 1461–1467.

15. ADA. *Directory of Dietetics Programs. 1977–1998.* The American Dietetic Association: Chicago; 1997.

16. Bogle, M.L., L. Balogun, J. Cassell, A. Catakis, H.J. Holler, and C. Flynn. "Achieving Excellence in Dietetic Practice: Certification of Specialists and Advanced-Level Practitioners." *J Am Diet Assoc* 93(1993): 149–150.

17. Bradley, R.T. "Fellow of the American Dietetic Association Credentialing Program: Development and Implementation of a Portfolio-Based Assessment." *J Am Diet Assoc* 96(1996): 513–517.

18. Personal communication with C. Reidy of the ADA/CDR, January 20, 2004.

19. Weddle, D.O., S.P. Himsburg, N. Collins, and R. Lewis. "The Professional Development Portfolio Process: Setting Goals for Credentialing." *J Am Diet Assoc* 102, no. 10(2002): 1439–1444.

20. Keim, K.S., G.E. Gates, and C.A. Johnson. "Dietetics Professionals Have a Positive Perception of Professional Development." *J Am Diet Assoc* 101, no. 7(2001): 820–824.

21. CDR/ADA. "CDR/ADA Adopts Policy on Appropriate Use of 'RD' and 'DTR' Credentials." *J Am Diet Assoc* 89(1989): 489–491.

CHAPTER 5

The Dietetics Professional

"Ethics in dietetics practice: complicated issues for a complicated time."[1]

OUTLINE

- Introduction
- Scope of Practice and Standards of Practice
- Ethical Practice
- Lifelong Professional Development
  - Lifelong Learning and Certification
  - Delivery of Learning
  - Informatics
  - Self-Responsibility for Learning
- Legal Basis of Practice
- Evidence-Based Practice
- Government Influence
- Summary

INTRODUCTION

Professional practice can be defined in several ways, first and foremost, as practice based on specialized learning and training and adherence to a code of ethical actions adopted by the group. Dietitians who develop a professional portfolio for registration status are familiar with the process involved, such as a plan for continued competence in practice with supporting goals and measures to reach the goals. The portfolio emphasis is on continued learning and self-monitoring, both distinguishing features of a professional.

A model for dietetics practice calls for a fluid and flexible framework for practice in dietetics.[2] The core of the profession is food and nutrition services for individuals, groups, and communities. The dietetics professional provides services through communication and collaboration with others by using management techniques, research, science, technology, and leadership skills.

SCOPE OF PRACTICE AND STANDARDS OF PRACTICE

In response to a need to provide guidance for members practicing in diverse roles in dietetics, the ADA appointed a task force in 2004 to develop a "Scope of Dietetics Practice" framework. This was completed in 2005 with further direction for usage by members following in 2006.[3,4] The framework provides a flexible decision-making structure by which practitioners can determine if specific activities fall within the scope of dietetics practice. Three broad areas are defined in the framework: foundation knowledge, evaluation resources, and decision aids.

The ADA first published guidelines for professional practice in 1998.[5] In 2003, these were replaced by the Standards of Professional Performance (SOPP) to more accurately describe their content and function.[6] Standards of Practice (SOP) also have been developed in many areas of dietetics practice. These are complementary documents. The SOP describes a skills competence level while the SOPP describes a competent level of behavior in the professional role. Together, they serve to describe the practice and performance of dietitians and dietetic technicians.

Standards are important for the following reasons:

- They promote safe, effective, and efficient food and nutrition services.
- They are based on evidence-based practice.
- They provide for improved health care and food and nutrition service-related outcomes.
- They ensure continuous quality improvement.

- They promote dietetics research, innovation, and practice development.
- They help the individual RD and DTR develop professionally.

Specific standards that have been developed in several areas of practice include: standards in nutrition care,[7] diabetes care,[8] oncology,[9] nutrition support,[10] behavioral health care,[11] management,[12] the education of dietetics practitioners,[13] sports dietetics,[14] and consultation.[15]

In addition to becoming proficient in an area of practice and continually monitoring performance, there are related areas of knowledge and practice that support and enhance competence but are not usually evident in a job description. Specifically, the areas discussed in this chapter include ethical practice, lifelong professional development, the legal basis of practice, political awareness, and evidence-based practice.

ETHICAL PRACTICE

The Professional Code of Ethics[16] is the guiding document for ethical practice in dietetics. The framework in which such policies are developed is the hallmark of an effective value structure that includes the following:[17]

- Guiding values and commitments are sensible and clearly communicated.
- Organizational leaders are personally committed, credible, and willing to take action on the values they espouse.
- Values are integrated into the normal channels of management decision making and are reflected in the organization's critical activities.
- The organization's systems and structures support and enforce its values.
- Managers throughout the organization have the decision-making skill, knowledge, and competencies needed to make ethically sound decisions on a day-to-day basis.

In practice, situations arise at times in which it is not always clear what the ethical course of action should be. Ethical conflicts of interest and poorly conducted business practices are examples of how ethical conduct impacts dietetic practice.[18–20] Other ethical considerations include issues of confidentiality, promotion and endorsement of products, and recognition of professional judgment.

In clinical practice, activities relating to dispensing dietary supplementation advice and conducting online counseling and consultation make it important to be familiar with laws and regulations as well as the code of ethics in order to avoid liability risk.[21] Other instances in which ethical conduct must be considered are disclosure of confidential information, accepting gifts, discussing patients, charting, or giving information about prices or salaries. In such cases, open discussion with a supervisor or

Table 5-1. Suggested Ethical Deliberative Process

1. Clarify the moral question—the first statement of the moral problem.
2. Re-create the context
   a. Gather data
   b. Relevant facts
   c. Relevant values
3. Name stakeholders and their relationships.
4. Identify ways of ethical thinking used by the stakeholders.
   a. Rules thinking—doing what is right by following the rules
   b. Roles thinking—being true to self and your sense of virtue
   c. Goals thinking—producing good outcomes regardless of rules
5. Determine practical limits to the situation: policies, laws, standards, and codes.
6. Balance a client's beliefs and preferences with his or her best interests.
7. Respect advance directives.
8. Assume a client has decisional capacity.
9. If not, select a substitute decisionmaker if necessary.
10. Restate the ethical problem.
11. Search for possible options.
12. Test various options. Check through each option for:
    a. rules—is it right?
    b. roles—can I feel good about this?
    c. goals—what good will it do?
13. Justify the option selected for recommendation.
    a. Keep the client's best interest at the center of options.
    b. Provide a description of what will likely happen and provide a clear action.
    c. Plan for each option recommended—suggestions of practical pathways.

Source: American Dietetic Association. "Position of the American Dietetic Association: Ethical and Legal Issues in Nutrition, Hydration, and Feeding." *J Am Diet Assoc* 102, no. 5(2002): 716–726.

trusted peers before action is the best course to follow. A personal code of conduct that espouses integrity, fairness, and a sense of always wanting to do "the right thing" helps make difficult decisions about ethical questions easier. The manager or leader assists in developing organization practices and policies that promote ethical practice. Such policies set the ethical standards for purchasing, financial management, patient care issues, information provided to patients and clients, and so on. The manager or leader sets an example for ethical behavior built on openness and trust. Resources for decision-making ethical dilemmas in dietetics are discussed by Holler.[22]

Increasingly, electronic communications involving the transmission of information on listservs and electronic health records demand ethical decision making.[23,24] Dietitians are also obligated to follow ethical standards when writing for the popular press.[25] An ethical deliberation process is shown in Table 5-1.

The ADA Code of Ethics for the Profession of Dietetics has been revised and adapted by the ADA and CDR as a voluntary enforceable code of ethics. This code challenges all members to uphold ethical principles. The process of enforcement includes a system to deal with any complaint about members and credentialed practitioners. The Ethics Committee is responsible for enforcing the code and educating members and the public about the ethical principles to be followed.[26]

LIFELONG PROFESSIONAL DEVELOPMENT

The Center for Professional Development in the ADA coordinates and offers many activities designed to support all food and nutrition professionals in continual building of their knowledge and skills through multidisciplinary activities, enhanced technology, and programming. Examples are the annual Food and Nutrition Conference and Exposition (FNCE); training programs for specialty certification; and conferences and events, including sessions at FNCE conducted by the dietetic practice groups. Distance learning opportunities are also offered through teleseminars and Webinars. In addition, group and individual self-study is available.

An initiative implemented in 2003 set forth a plan to improve compensation levels through professional development activities by the association and its members.[27] The "Performance, Proficiency, and Value Plan" set forth the following two goals:

1. The ADA invests in various approaches to close the gaps between performance, proficiency, and value for the profession of dietetics and identifies strategies to do so.
2. Members adopt various approaches to enhance personal value.

Many positive benefits have come from the undertaking, both professionally and through increased compensation levels (see Chapter 2).

The importance of professional development is also emphasized by Dodd[28] and Dowling,[29] both of whom address personal responsibility for professional performance. Fuhrman[30] recommends strategies to increase the credibility and visibility in clinical dietetics by being open to earning opportunities, being assertive, justifying recommendations, maintaining competency and skills in one's area of practice, and enjoying what one does!

Lifelong Learning and Certification

Because lifelong learning is so important to professionalism in practice, continuing professional education (CPE) has always been the cornerstone of certification of the dietitian. The Professional Development Resource Center at the ADA provides many opportunities for lifelong learning and each state provides continuing education through state meetings, conferences, and other events. Self-study courses, graduate degrees, and publishing are further ways of gaining credit for continued learning and maintenance of registration.

The Professional Development Portfolio (PDP) is the individual plan submitted by each dietitian outlining his or her plan for learning that qualifies for continuing education credit. The steps required in the plan are:

1. The individual reflects on his or her practice, including strengths, needed improvements, identification of interests and trends, and then establishes short- and long-term goals.
2. The individual conducts a learning needs assessment by identifying the knowledge and skills needed to achieve the goals and define the level of CPE necessary to meet the goals.
3. The individual develops a plan to meet the goals through participation in learning activities. The plan is submitted to the CDR for approval.

4. The plan is implemented through continuing professional education.
5. The outcomes are evaluated by the individual.

Duyff[31] points to several characteristics of the lifelong learner: ongoing curiosity, motivation to learn, confidence in the ability to learn from others and to share knowledge, the willingness to make and learn from mistakes, persistence, flexible thinking, and diligence required to gather adequate information before drawing conclusions. Self-awareness, self-monitoring, positive "self-talk," and reflection are also needed. Adult learners succeed most often when learning is self-directed, practical, experience-based, interactive, applied, and individualized.

Delivery of Learning

Food and nutrition professionals use a variety of methods to continually build their knowledge and skills. The range of learning opportunities is greater than ever considering the many advancements in technology that allow individual study as well as group learning and interaction. For instance, teleconferencing today replaces many former face-to-face meetings, thus saving travel and related costs. Networking through social network sites is fast becoming a way for dietetic professionals to connect with and learn from others with similar interests and concerns.[32,33]

Technologies often used in distance education are *synchronous* (participants meet together) or *asynchronous* (participant access course materials on their own). Examples of synchronous methods are individual and conference calls, videoconferencing, and web conferencing. Asynchronous methods include audiocassette, e-mail, message board forums, print materials, voicemail, fax, CDs, and videocassette. Distance education courses are offered in several ways: by correspondence through regular mail; through the Internet, either synchronously or asynchronously; through telecourses in which content is delivered by radio or television; CD-ROM instruction in which the student interacts with computer content stored in the file; pocket/mobile learning through mobile devices or wireless service; and integrated learning through in-group instruction with a distance learning curriculum.

Online video and streaming video have proven to be a very effective ways of communicating nutrition messages.[34] Switt[35] offers suggestions for creating and managing a Web site by offering unique, original content; registering with search engines; and developing a newsletter.

Informatics

Informatics is the fast-growing area of electronic support for using and managing information. Health informatics is described by the Department of Health and Human Services as the intersections of information science, computer science, and health care.[36] Health information tools include electronic media, clinical guidelines, formal medical terminologies, and information and communication systems. The medical and nursing professions have taken the lead in use of the technology, most directly in the development of electronic health records.[37]

Nutrition informatics is defined as "the effective retrieval, organization, storage, and optimum use of information, data, and knowledge for food and nutrition-related problem solving and decision making. Informatics is supported by the use of information standards, information processes, and information technology."[38] In 2007, a Nutrition Information Work Group was appointed to examine the state of nutrition information across the practice of dietitians.[39] A survey was designed to determine the extent of member utilization of this technology. It was found that while dietitians use e-mail and the Internet extensively, the concept of nutrition informatics is new and not well understood by dietitians but that there is a great deal of interest in its use.

A national undertaking in 2004 set a goal of an electronic health record for every American by 2014.[40] The initiative was spearheaded by the Department of Health and Human Services Information Initiative. The dietetic profession is a part of this national effort, making it imperative that a concerted effort is made to prepare practitioners for the use of nutrition information aligned with the broad field of medicine, health, and nursing information.

Self-Responsibility for Learning

Self-direction in learning is the ability to engage in educational activities without external reinforcement. Individuals who do so embody some or all of the following characteristics:

- Willingness to change
- Ability to identify weaknesses or shortcomings
- Ability to capitalize on strengths and passions
- Ability to experience learning from constructive criticism

- Willingness to participate in all forms of learning
- Willingness to try new techniques for learning
- Willingness to invest one's time and money in learning
- Willingness to find a mentor or become one
- Volunteering in organizations and groups
- Sharing learning by applying concepts and discussing with others
- Providing feedback to instructors, mentors, and supervisors
- Assuming individual responsibility for learning
- Allowing the possibility of new careers, life oaths, and experiences

Besides maintaining and improving professional competence, there are other reasons why practitioners participate in continuing education activities and why there may be deterrents to doing so. Several reasons and deterrents are shown in Table 5-2.

To determine the types of learning experiences that most benefit an individual, several questions may be posed for self-examination of needs (Table 5-3).

Table 5-2. Factors Influencing Continuing Professional Education

Reasons for participation in Continuing Professional Education:
· Professional development and improvement
· Professional service
· Collegial learning and interaction
· Professional commitment and reflection
· Personal benefits and job security

Deterrents in predicting participation in Continuing Professional Education:
· Disengagement and apathy for learning or career
· Costs
· Family
· Failure to see the worth or benefit
· Lack of quality in offerings
· Demands of work constraints

Source: Petrillo, T. "Lifelong Learning Goals: Individual Steps That Propel the Profession of Dietetics." *J Am Diet Assoc* 103, no. 3(2003): 298–300.

Table 5-3. Questions to Determine Self Needs

What kind of learning is needed to improve performance in your current job?

Analyze your current job. Talk with supervisors and discuss how to change or improve your current job.

What is your capacity for learning and growth in a new job?

What transferable skills do you possess for a new career path?

What new skills are required for you to be qualified to contribute in a new job?

What are your personal interests?

What career paths did you once consider?

What leisure time interests do you enjoy?

What type of a learning experience is most favorable to you and why?

What related learning opportunities lie just beyond your field of practice?

What skill sets are important to your employer?

Sources: Data from Davis, J.R. *Toolbox for Reflection and Developing an Action Learning Plan: Managing Your Own.* Berrett-Koehler Publisher, 2000 (10).

Petrillo, T. "Lifelong Learning Goals: Individual Steps that Propel the Profession of Dietetics." *J Am Diet Assoc* 103, no. 3(2003): 298–300.

LEGAL BASIS OF PRACTICE

The practice of dietetics is directly affected by many laws and regulations that must be followed in order to avoid legal consequences. Fortunately, as Derelian[41] points out, almost all disputes that include a dietitian would be of a civil nature, such as contract breaches or negligence. Busey[42] indicates that dietitians increasingly may become parties to lawsuits considering the number of RDs who go into private practice and the fact that RDs play important roles in the healthcare process. He gives suggestions regarding the types of lawsuits in which a dietitian may become involved and discusses steps in the process when lawsuits occur. Busey[43] further points out that if the terminology used in documentation of patient care is subject to more than one interpretation, this could become a legally disputed issue in a lawsuit. An example is the use of the word "inadequate" in describing patient progress as it could denote negligence.

The increasing trend toward greater use of electronic technology such as in telehealth or telemedicine in which a dietitian may be a participant is another area in which legal questions may arise.[44] Examples of practice issues that may apply are licensure, facility certification and accreditation, reimbursement and Medicare Part B issues, and professional liability issuance.

All dietitians are strongly encouraged to carry personal liability insurance for protection against malpractice or when issues such as have been described occur.

EVIDENCE-BASED PRACTICE

Evidence-based practice (EBP) is increasingly viewed as necessary for the best outcomes in all areas of dietetic practice. Evidence-based medicine is a model of clinical decision making that uses a "systematic process to integrate the best research-based evidence with clinical expertise and patient values to answer a question about a patient's plan of care in order to optimize outcomes."[45] In dietetics, EBP can be described as a process by which the best available data are consulted to make decisions, followed by evaluation of the outcome of these decisions.[46] Dietitians need to incorporate evidence-based practice into all activities and decisions, payment for services may be dependent on outcomes, because change in practice is constant, and this approach ensures that decisions are sound.[47,48] Evidence-based practice is especially vital in all clinical and patient-related activities and is critical in justifying reimbursement for medical nutrition therapy. By applying this process, dietitians are able to successfully compete in the healthcare environment where positive outcomes, proven efficiency, cost effectiveness, and sharing of outcomes are important.[49] The healthcare manager, who may be the dietitian in charge of a unit, is often the catalyst for assuring that evidence-based information is integrated into healthcare management decisions.[50]

A study in 2005[51] reported that of 500 randomly selected dietitians, most had favorable opinions of the evidence-based research process but many were not prepared to use the procedure. Fortunately, the ADA now provides a valuable resource to members through the Evidence Analysis Library (EAL) available at www.adaevidencelibrary.com. Through the EAL process outlined, professionals can stay up-to-date on the technical research being done in all areas of dietetics. A variety of resources are offered, including evidence summaries of the major research on a given topic, bibliographies, and conclusion statements with an evaluation of the strength of the evidence.[52]

Straus and Haynes[53] provide a clear guide for appraising resources for evidence-based information (see Table 5-4). They point out that evidence must be balanced with the client's values and preferences for optimal shared decision making, and that information resources must be reliable, relevant, and readable.

Table 5-4. Guide for Appraising Resources for Evidence-Based Information

Methods and quality of information

· How was the resource compiled?

· Were explicit criteria for seeking and appraising evidence described and were they adhered to?

· How is the resource maintained?

Rating scale for methods and quality of information

0 No evidence cited

1 Evidence is cited but there are no explicit criteria for the selection or the evaluation of the content; the election of content suggests lack of consistent evidence standards.

2 Evidence is cited and there are explicit criteria for the selection or evaluation of the content, or both; the selection of content suggests lack of adherence to these evidence standards.

3 Evidence is cited but there are no explicit criteria for the selection or evaluation of the content; the selection of content suggest adherence to some evidence standards.

4 Evidence is cited and there are explicit criteria for the selection or evaluation of the content, or both; the selection of content suggests some adherence to evidence standards.

5 Evidence is cited and there are explicit criteria for the selection and evaluation of the content; the selection of content suggests adherence to evidence standards most of the time.

Clinical usefulness

· Did the resource provide clinically useful answers?

· How did you use this resource?

· Was it easy to use?

· Were the answers easily accessible and readable within a few minutes?

· Will you use this resource?

· If so, when and how?

(continues)

Table 5-4. Guide for Appraising Resources for Evidence-Based Information *(continued)*

Rating scale for clinical usefulness

0 Not useful clinically

1 Clinically useful answers are rarely available and are not easily accessible or readable within a few minutes.

2 Clinically useful answers are available some of the time but are not easily accessible or readable within a few minutes.

3 Clinically useful answers are available some of the time and are easily accessible and readable within a few minutes.

4 Clinically useful answers are available most of the time but are not easily accessible or readable within a few minutes.

5 Clinically useful answers are available most of the time and are easily accessible and readable within a few minutes.

Details on specific resources

Evidence-based medical texts

The following points could be used as a minimum checklist:

· Does the resource provide an explicit statement about the type of evidence on which any statements or recommendations are based? Did the authors adhere to these criteria? For example, claims about effectiveness of an intervention might be accompanied by a statement about either the level of evidence (which would need to be defined somewhere in the text) or a statement about the exact type of evidence (e.g., "there have been three randomized controlled trials").

· Was there an explicit and adequate search for this evidence? For example, a search for evidence about an intervention might have started with a look for adequate systematic reviews. If this was done, it might be followed by a search of the Cochrane Central Register of Controlled Trials.

· Is there quantification of the results? For example, statements about diagnostic accuracy should contain measures of accuracy such as sensitivity and specificity.

The minimum criteria for an evidence-based resource would be adherence to the first point. Better resources should also address the other two points.

Meta-resources (e.g., listings or search engines for other resources)

· These resources should provide an explicit statement about the selection criteria for inclusion in the listing. Better resources should also include a descriptive review such as that described in the three points for evidence-based medical texts.

Source: Straus, S. and R.B. Haynes. "Managing Evidence-Based Knowledge: The Need for Reliable, Relevant, and Readable Resources." *CMAJ* 180, no. 9(2009): 942–945.

GOVERNMENT INFLUENCE

Dietitians in all areas of practice are influenced by actions of governmental bodies because the accreditation of programs and credentialing of professionals have the backing and authority of a governmental body. For example, state licensure is enacted by state legislative action.

Congress and state legislatures enact laws regarding health care, the reimbursement for those working in health care, and the practitioner qualifications. The Food and Drug Administration (FDA) regulates the safety of drugs and foods, and therefore what is allowed on the market. Similarly, the U.S. Department of Agriculture (USDA) regulates meat and poultry products on the market. The U.S. Dietary Guidelines for Americans are issued by the Department of Health and Human Services (DHHS) and the USDA jointly every 5 years. The USDA provides numerous educational materials for use in adhering to the recommendations of the Guidelines such as the MyPyramid and the Healthy Eating Index (HEI). Regulations pertaining to child nutrition programs, that is, school breakfast and lunch programs, summer feeding programs, and daycare, are provided by the USDA. The Special Supplemental Nutrition Program for Women, Infants, and Children Program (WIC), and the Supplemental Nutrition Assistance Program (SNAP) are administered through the USDA. The Academy of Sciences, through the Institute of Medicine and the Food and Nutrition Board, publishes nutrient intake guides for the population. Other governmental agencies issue guidelines for staffing and procedures in all healthcare institutions receiving federal or state monies, one example being the Joint Commission on Accreditation of Healthcare Organizations (JCAHO).

Each year, the Legislative and Public Policy Committee of ADA, under the direction of the Board of Directors, establishes policy priorities based on member and association interests and legislation under consideration at the national level. The priority areas in which the ADA works from year to year include food and food safety, healthcare reform, health literacy and nutrition advancement, medical nutrition therapy, aging, child nutrition, Medicaid and Medicare, nutrition monitoring and research, obesity, and healthy weight management.[54]

SUMMARY

The professional dietitian is one who is competent in practice and continually participates in ongoing education. Knowledge and skills go hand in hand with personal qualities and practices, including ethical practice, awareness of government influence, understanding of the legal basis of practice, and incorporating the concept of evidence-based activities into professional practice. As the voice of authority in food and nutrition, the dietitian is a professional in every sense of the term.

DEFINITIONS

Ethics. Moral concepts of correctness and honor.

Evidence-Based. Action based on best data and evaluation of outcomes.

Legislative Action. The enactment of laws by Congress or a state legislature.

Profession. An occupation that involves specialized knowledge and training in which members subscribe to group beliefs and practices.

Public Policy. Course of action by a government entity for its people.

Regulation. A written directive that implements and puts a law into effect.

REFERENCES

1. Gallagher, A. "Ethics in Dietetics Practice: Complicated Issues for a Complicated Time." *J Am Diet Assoc* 99, no. 11(1999): 1348.
2. Commission on Accreditation of Dietetics Education. *Accreditation Handbook.* The American Dietetic Association: Chicago; 2002, p. 9.
3. Maillet, J., J. Skates, and E. Pritchett. "American Dietetic Association: Scope of Dietetics Practice Framework." *J Am Diet Assoc* 105, no. 4(2005): 634–640.
4. Viscosan, B. and J. Switt. "Undertaking and Using the Scope of Dietetics Practice Framework: A Step-Wise Approach." *J Am Diet Assoc* 106, no. 3(2006): 459–463.
5. ADA. "The American Dietetic Association Standards of Professional Practice for Dietetics Professionals." *J Am Diet Assoc* 98, no. 1(1998): 83–87.
6. Kieselhorst, K.J., J. Skates, and E. Pritchett. "American Dietetic Association: Standards of Practice in Nutrition Care and Updated Standards of Professional Performance." *J Am Diet Assoc* 105, no. 4(2005): 641–645.
7. The American Dietetic Association Quality Management Committee. "American Dietetic Association Revised 2008 Standards of Practice for Registered Dietitians in Nutrition Care; Standards of Professional Performance for Registered Dietitians; Standards of Practice for Dietetic Technicians, Registered, in Nutrition Care; and Standards of Professional Performance for Dietetic Technicians, Registered." *J Am Diet Assoc* 108, no. 9(2008): 1538–1542.
8. Kulkarni, K., J.L. Boucher, A. Daly, C.S. Slavin, B.T. Silvers, J.O. Maillet, and E. Pritchett. "American Dietetic Association: Standards of Practice and Standards of Professional Performance for Registered Dietitians (Generalist, Specialty, and Advanced) in Diabetes Care." *J Am Diet Assoc* 105, no. 5(2005): 819–824.
9. Robien, K., R. Levin, E. Pritchett, and M. Otto. "American Dietetic Association: Standards of Practice and Standards of Professional Performance for Registered Dietitians (Generalist, Specialty, and Advanced) in Oncology Nutrition Care." *J Am Diet Assoc* 106, no. 6(2006): 946–951.

10. The Joint Standards Task Force of A.S.P.E.N. and the American Dietetic Association Dietitians in Nutrition Support Dietetic Practice Group. "American Society for Parenteral and Enteral Nutrition and the American Dietetic Association: Standards of Practice and Standards of Professional Performance for Registered Dietitians (Generalist, Specialty, and Advanced) in Nutrition Support." *J Am Diet Assoc* 107, no. 10(2007): 1815–1822.

11. Emerson, M., P. Kerr, M.D.C. Soler, T. A. Girard, R. Hoffinger, E. Pritchett, and M. Otto. "American Dietetic Association Standards of Practice and Standards of Professional Performance for Registered Dietitians (Generalist, Specialty, and Advanced) in Behavioral Health Care." *J Am Diet Assoc* 106, no. 6(2006): 608–613.

12. Puckett, R.P., M. Barkley, G. Dixon, K. Egan, C. Koch, T. Malone, J. Scott-Smith, B. Sheridan, and M. Theis. "American Dietetic Association: Standards of Professional Performance for Registered Dietitians (Generalist and Advanced) in Management of Food and Nutrition Systems." *J Am Diet Assoc* 109, no. 3(2009): 540–552.

13. Anderson, J.A., K. Kennedy-Hagan, M.R. Stieber, D.S. Hollingsworth, K. Kattelmann, C. L. Stein Arnold, and B.M. Egan. "Dietetics Educators of Practitioners and American Dietetic Association Standards of Professional Performance for Registered Dietitians (Generalist, Specialty/Advanced) in Education of Dietetics Practitioners." *J Am Diet Assoc* 109, no. 4(2009): 747–754.

14. Steinmuller, P.L., N.L. Meyer, L.K. Fruskall, M.N. Manore, N.R. Rodriguez, M. Macedonio, R.L. Bird, and J.R. Berning. "American Dietetic Association Standards of Practice and Standards of Professional performance for Registered Dietitians (Generalist, Specialty, Advanced) in Sports Dietetics." *J Am Diet Assoc* 109, no. 3(2009): 544–551.

15. Vogelzang, J.L. and L.L. Roth-Yousey. "Standards of Professional Practice: Measuring the Beliefs and Realities of Consultant Dietitians in Health Care Facilities." *J Am Diet Assoc* 102, no. 4(2001): 473–480.

16. American Dietetic Association/Commission on Dietetic Registration. "Code of Ethics for the Profession of Dietetics." *J Am Diet Assoc* 109, no. 8(2009): 1461–1467.

17. Paine, L.S. "Managing for Organizational Integrity." *Harvard Business Review* 72(1994): 106–117.

18. Waynack, M.H. "Ethical Conflicts of Interest." *J Am Diet Assoc* 103, no. 5(2003): 555–557.

19. Fornari, A. "Professional Boundary Issues in Practice." *J Am Diet Assoc* 103, no. 3(2003): 380.

20. Fornari, A. "Characteristics of Ethical Issues Versus Poor Business Practices." *J Am Diet Assoc* 103, no. 10(2002): 1380–1381.

21. Fuhrman, M.P. "Issues Facing Dietetics Professionals: Challenges and Opportunities." *J Am Diet Assoc* 102, no. 11(2002): 1618–1620.

22. Holler, H. "Resources for Ethical Dilemmas in Dietetics." *J Am Diet Assoc* 100, no. 5(2000): 515.

23. Castle, D. and R. DeBusk. "The Electronic Health Record: Genetic Information and Patient Privacy." *J Am Diet Assoc* 108, no. 8(2008): 1372–1374.

24. American Dietetic Association 2005–2006 Ethics Committee. "Ethics Opinion: Conflicting Interest Disclosure on Listservs." *J Am Diet Assoc* 106, no. 7(2006): 1025–1026.

25. American Dietetic Association 2005–2006 Ethics Committee. "Ethics Opinion: The RD and DTR Are Obligated to Follow Ethical Standards When Writing for the Popular Press." *J Am Diet Assoc* 107, no. 12(2007): 2052–2054.

26. See note 16.

27. American Dietetic Association. 2005–2006 Ethics Committee. "Performance, Proficiency, and Value of the Dietetics Professional: An Update." *J Am Diet Assoc* 103, no. 10(2003): 1376–1379.

28. Dodd, J.L. "Look Before You Leap—But Do Leap!" *J Am Diet Assoc* 99, no. 4(1999): 422–425.

29. Dowling, R. "Role Expansion for Dietetics Professionals." *J Am Diet Assoc* 96, no. 10(1996): 1001–1002.

30. Fuhrman, M.P. "Issues Facing Dietetics Professionals: Challenges and Opportunities." *J Am Diet Assoc* 102, no. 11(2002): 1618–1620.

31. Duyff, R.L. "The Value of Lifelong Learning: Key Element in Professional Career Development." *J Am Diet Assoc* 99, no. 5(1999): 538–543.

32. Graham, L.K. "What Is Social Networking? And How Do I Get Clued in to LinkedIn?" *J Am Diet Assoc* 109, no. 1(2009): 184.

33. Brown, D. "Networking Moves Online." *J Am Diet Assoc* 109, no. 2(2009): 210–211.

34. Lane, M. "Streaming Soon to a Computer Near You: How Online Video Will Change Media (and Maybe Your Practice) Forever." *ADA Times* 5, no. 1(2007): 12–15.

35. Switt, J.T. "Drawing Attention to Your Web Site." *J Am Diet Assoc* 108, no. 1(2008): 20.

36. U.S. Department of Health and Human Services. "Health Information Technology." www.busus.gov (Accessed April 6, 2009).

37. Hoggle, L.B., M.A. Michael, S.M. Houston, and E.J. Ayers. "Nutrition Informatics." *J Am Diet Assoc* 108, no. 1(2008): 134–139.

38. Yadrick, M.M. "Informatics: A Word We Need to Know." President's Page. *J Am Diet Assoc* 108, no. 1(2008): 1976.

39. Ayres, E. "ADA Nutrition Informatics Member Survey: Results and Future Steps." *J Am Diet Assoc* 108, no. 11(2008): 1822–1826.

40. Hoggle, L.B., M.A. Michael, S.M. Houston, and E.J. Ayres. "Electronic Health Record: Where Does Nutrition Fit In?" *J Am Diet Assoc* 106, no. 10(2006): 1688–1695.

41. Derelian, D. "Dietetics: Legalities, Ethics, and Eccentricities." *J Am Diet Assoc* 100, no. 5(2000): 519–523.

42. Busey, J.C. "Help! I've Just Been Served with a Lawsuit." *J Am Diet Assoc* 109, no. 4(2009): 600–605.

43. Busey, J.C. "Use of the Word *Inadequate*—A Legal Perspective." *J Am Diet Assoc* 108, no. 6(2008): 935–936.

44. Busey, J.C. "Telehealth—Opportunities and Pitfalls." *J Am Diet Assoc* 108, no. 8(2008): 1296–1301.

45. Shanklin, C. "Evidence-Based Practice: Practice Based on Evidence, Right?" *ADA Times* 1, no. 3(2003): 1,3.

46. Blumberg-Kason, S. "Evidence-Based Nutrition Practice Guidelines: A Valuable Resource in the Evidence Analysis Library." *J Am Diet Assoc* 106, no. 12(2006): 1935–1936.

47. Vaughan, L.A. and C.K. Manning. "Meeting the Challenges of Dietetics Practice with Evidence-Based Decisions." *J Am Diet Assoc* 104, no. 2(2004): 282–284.

48. Franz, M.J. "The Lenna Frances Cooper Memorial Lecture—The Future of Clinical Dietetics: Evidence, Outcomes, and Reimbursement." *J Am Diet Assoc* 103, no. 8(2003): 977–981.

49. Smith, R. "Expanding Medical Nutrition Therapy: An Argument for Evidence-Based Practices." *J Am Diet Assoc* 103, no. 3(2003): 313–314.

50. Smith, K.P.D. and J. Woods. "The Healthcare Manager as Catalyst for Evidence-Based Practice: Changing the Healthcare Environment and Changing Experience." *Healthcare Papers* 300, no. 3(2003): 54–57.

51. Byham-Gray, L.D., J.D. Gilbride, B. Dixon, and F.K. Stage. "Evidence-Based Practice: What Are Dietitian's Perceptions, Attitudes, and Knowledge?" *J Am Diet Assoc* 105, no. 10(2005): 1574–1581.

52. See Note 51.

53. Straus, S. and R.B. Haynes. "Managing Evidence-Based Knowledge: The Need for Reliable, Relevant and Readable Resources." *CMAJ* 180, no. 9(2009): 942–945.

54. ADA. "Legislative Priorities." www.eatright.org (Accessed April 5, 2009).

Part III
Areas of Practice

CHAPTER 6

The Dietitian in Clinical Practice

"The dietetic practitioner interacts with complex beings who eat food rather than nutrients. The psychosocial aspects of diet modification may therefore determine ultimate clinical usefulness and ethical practice."[1]

OUTLINE

- Introduction
- Employment Settings of Clinical Dietitians
- Organization of Clinical Nutrition Services
- Responsibilities in Clinical Dietetics
  - Nutrition Care Process and Model
  - Medical Nutrition Therapy
  - Standards of Practice
- The Clinical Nutrition Service Team
  - Clinical Nutrition Manager or Chief Clinical Dietitian
  - Clinical Dietitian
  - Dietetic Technicians
  - Dietetic Assistants
- Clinical Dietetics Outlook
  - Healthcare Reform
  - Public Opinion Survey
  - Newer Communication Methods
  - Clinical Privileging
- Summary

INTRODUCTION

The discipline of clinical dietetics originated in 1899 when "dietitian" was defined by the American Home Economics Association as "individuals with a knowledge of food who provide diet therapy for the medical profession." Until 1917, dietitians were affiliated with this association, but after 1917 they belonged to the newly formed American Dietetic Association.[2]

The earliest dietitians worked primarily in hospitals or were associated with food assistance programs. During the 1930s and 1940s, dietitians became involved either in food production and food service or in the planning and provision of diets for special medical needs. The title "therapeutic dietitian" was used to describe the person who provided food for medical reasons, such as the prevention of a nutrient deficiency or to help with the treatment of disease.[3] Examples of early diet therapy are the Sippy diet that used milk and cream to treat ulcers and the Kempner rice diet to treat hypertension; each was named for the physician who designed it.

As the dietitian's role in the hospital became one of providing specialized care and modifying diets to treat various medical conditions, the title "clinical dietitians" replaced the former titles.

In the early 1970s, reports of widespread malnutrition among hospitalized patients helped to increase the visibility of clinical dietitians.[4] Clinical dietitians began to take a more active role in screening and monitoring the provision of nutrition support. Development of individual nutrition care plans became important functions of clinical dietitians. As the role of diet in the etiology of chronic diseases became better defined, clinical dietitians began to spend a greater proportion of their time participating in the prevention of diseases such as heart disease, cancer, and diabetes.

EMPLOYMENT SETTINGS OF CLINICAL DIETITIANS

In 2009, 85 percent of the most recent survey of RDs and DTRs reported they were currently employed in dietetics.[5] In fact, this high percentage of dietitians and dietetic technicians who were working in the field of dietetics reflects the diversity of job opportunities. Tables 6-1 and 6-2 show the primary employment settings of dietitians. Fifty-six percent of RDs and 57 percent of DTRs were employed in the clinical areas of practice. These findings and earlier membership surveys with similar findings indicate stability in these employment areas.

The primary areas of clinical practice are:

1. Acute care/inpatient
   a. Hospitals
2. Ambulatory care
   a. hospital outpatient departments
   b. clinics
   c. outpatient care centers
3. Long-term care
   a. nursing homes
   b. assisted living facilities
   c. Alzheimer's disease units

Table 6-1. Practice Area, Primary Position

	RDs (%)	DTRs (%)
Clinical nutrition—acute care/inpatient	30	39
Clinical nutrition—ambulatory care	17	1
Clinical nutrition—long-term care	9	17
Community	11	10
Food and nutrition management	12	19
Consultation and business	8	2
Education and research	7	2

Base: 8115 practicing RDs and DTRs.

Source: American Dietetic Association. Compensation and Benefits Survey of the Dietetics Profession 2009. www.eatright.org.

Table 6-2. Highest Incidence Positions—RDs

	RDs (%)
Clinical dietitian	16
Outpatient dietitian, general	4
Outpatient dietitian, specialist—diabetes	5
Outpatient dietitian, specialist—renal	4
Clinical dietitian, long-term care	9
Women, infants, and children nutritionist	5
Director of food and nutrition services	4
Private practice dietitian—patient/client nutrition care	2

Source: American Dietetic Association. Compensation and Benefits Survey of the Dietetics Profession 2009. www.eatright.org.

ORGANIZATION OF CLINICAL NUTRITION SERVICES

Clinical nutrition services may be organized in a variety of ways, depending on the setting. Clinical nutrition services in most hospitals are managed by a clinical nutrition manager, the director of clinical nutrition, or the chief clinical dietitian (Figure 6-1a). Typically, the chief clinical dietitian reports to an individual whose primary responsibilities are food service and the financial management of the entire food and nutrition department. In some instances, clinical dietetics may be organized as a separate department that reports to an executive or administrator with other patient care responsibilities such as nursing or pharmacy (Figure 6-1b). There are advantages and disadvantages to both types of organization. Combining clinical nutrition with food services can facilitate communication regarding patient food choices and menus. By contrast, having clinical nutrition as a separate department may increase visibility as an important patient care service unit distinct from food service.

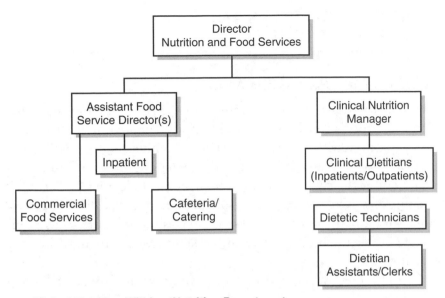

a. Clinical Nutrition Within a Nutrition Department

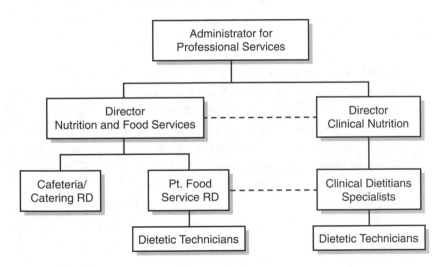

b. Clinical Nutrition Within a Separate Department

FIGURE 6-1a AND b. Examples of Nutrition and Food Service Organizational Charts.

Sources: Example a is courtesy of The Methodist Hospital, Houston, Texas. Example b is courtesy of Nutrition Center, Arkansas Children's Hospital, Little Rock, Arkansas.

RESPONSIBILITIES IN CLINICAL DIETETICS

Nutrition Care Process and Model

The Quality Management Committee of the ADA developed a nutrition care process (NCP) and model that was adopted by the House of Delegates in 2003.[6] The purpose of the planning model was "for implementation and dissemination to the dietetics profession and the association for the enhancement of the practice of dietetics."[7] The NCP is defined as systematic problem-solving methods that dietetic professionals use to critically think and make decisions to address nutrition-related problems and to provide safe and effective quality nutrition care (Figure 6-2).

In 2008, a review and update of the process was undertaken following a survey of ADA groups experienced in using the NCP.[8] The process (now referred to as the nutrition care process and model (NCPM) included revisions in the original model and defined the functions under each step as follows:

1. **Nutrition Assessment.** In step 1, a systematic approach to collect, record, and interpret relevant data from patients, clients, family members, caregivers, and other individual groups is undertaken. Examples of the type of data collected are: food- and nutrition-related history, anthropometric measurements, biochemical data, medical tests and procedures, nutrition-focused physical examination findings, and client history.

2. **Nutrition Diagnosis.** Nutrition professionals identify and label existing nutrition problems they are responsible for treating independently. The determination for continuation of care follows this step.

3. **Nutrition Intervention.** Action is taken with the intent of changing a nutrition-related behavior, risk factor, environmental condition, or aspect of health status. This entails writing a plan of care, collaborating with the patient or client to identify goals of the interaction, and partnering with the patient and other caregivers to carry out the plan.

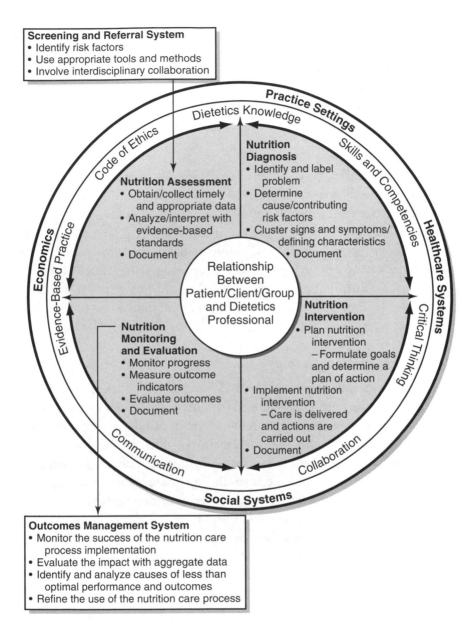

FIGURE 6-2. The ADA Nutrition Care Process and Model.

Source: Lacey, K. and E. Pritchett. "Nutrition Care Process and Model." *J Am Diet Assoc* 103, no. 8(2003): 1061–1071.

4. **Nutrition Monitoring and Evaluation.** In this final step, the amount of progress is identified and whether the goals and expected outcomes are being met. Three steps are involved:
   a. Monitor progress.
   b. Measure the outcomes.
   c. Evaluate the outcomes by comparing to earlier status or reference standards.

A standardized language or set of terms is being developed to describe the results in each step of the NCPM.[9] The terms are from the International Dietetics and Nutrition Terminology (IDNT), under development by the ADA in order to facilitate the inclusion of RD activities in electronic health record-keeping, and also in policies, procedures, rules, and legislation. The use of such standardized reporting will primarily assist in documenting nutrition care in the medical record in a way that will refer to each of the four steps in the NCPM and highlight the role of nutrition in patient care.

Medical Nutrition Therapy

Medical nutrition therapy (MNT) was defined in 1995 by the ADA as: "the assessment of the nutritional status of patients with a condition, illness, or injury that puts them at risk."[10] This assessment includes review and analysis of the medical and diet history, laboratory values, and anthropometric measurements. Based on the assessment, nutrition applications most appropriate to manage the condition or treat the injury are chosen. These include diet modification, counseling, and specialized nutrition therapies.

A full history of the development of MNT, its importance in the national healthcare discussion, and the challenges presented to members of the ADA were discussed by the Government Relations office of the ADA in 2005.[11]

The rationale and justification for the successful passage of legislation extending MNT to other disease treatments depends, in large part, on the evidence that can be demonstrated regarding its beneficial effects.[12] Cost containment is a critical part of all healthcare reform measures and any new MNT programs will likely demand good scientific evidence of both its cost-effectiveness and efficacy. To this end, evidence-based outcomes research that documents the clinical effectiveness of MNT is all-important. Evidence-based practice (EBP), it follows, improves the quality of care and helps manage costs. By adopting EBP in providing MNT, RDs will use the best available evidence to provide therapy, in addition to their own clinical expertise and experience.

The ADA assists all dietitians by maintaining a library of resources, the Evidence Analysis Library (EAL), available online at www.adaevidence library.com. The EAL gathers the best, most current, and most relevant research on important questions in dietetics practice and is available at no cost to all ADA members.[13] The EAL offers evidence-based nutrition practice guidelines in areas such as lipid metabolism, adult weight management, and critical illnesses.

It should be noted that the nutrition care process is the broader, over-arching guide to a full spectrum of nutrition care, and medical nutrition therapy is a process for delivery of nutrition care. The NCP specifies the steps a dietitian would use in delivering the therapy, but also guides nutrition education and preventive nutrition care services.

Standards of Practice

The "Standards of Practice in Nutrition Care" describe the minimum expectations for competent nutrition care practice. The "Standards of Professional Performance," a companion document, describe the expectation for competent behavior in the nondirect patient or client nutrition care aspect of RD and DTR roles. Standards were updated in 2008.[14]

The four Standards of Practice (SOP) in nutrition care follow the steps in the nutrition care process. They are:

SOP 1. Nutrition Assessment
SOP 2. Nutrition Diagnoses
SOP 3. Nutrition Intervention
SOP 4. Nutrition Monitoring and Evaluation

The Standards of Professional Performance (SOPP) are the following;

SOPP 1. Provide quality service based on customer expectations and needs.
SOPP 2. Participate in and apply research to enhance practice.
SOPP 3. Effectively apply knowledge and communicate with others.
SOPP 4. Use resources effectively and efficiently.
SOPP 5. Systematically evaluate the quality of services and improve practice based on evaluation of results.
SOPP 6. Engage in lifelong learning.

Standards of Practice and Standards of Professional Performance for the dietetic technician are included in the same document (see reference 14).

THE CLINICAL NUTRITION SERVICE TEAM

Clinical nutrition services may be provided by a number of team members in healthcare facilities. Inpatient nutritional care in hospitals is usually the responsibility of persons in several positions: clinical nutrition managers or chief clinical dietitians, clinical dietitians, dietetic technicians, and dietetic assistants. Outpatient clinics and ambulatory care centers may use all four positions but are more likely to employ only clinical dietitians. Extended care facilities and physician offices may have clinical dietitians on staff; however, more often these facilities use a consulting dietitian to provide MNT for selected patients and clients. Consulting dietitians may be in private practice or part of a group practice.

Clinical Nutrition Manager or Chief Clinical Dietitian

The clinical nutrition manager or chief clinical dietitian is primarily responsible for directing the activities of clinical dietitians, dietetic technicians, and dietetic assistants. Major tasks performed include developing and managing budgets for the clinical area, hiring clinical nutrition employees, evaluating employee job performance, providing in-service and on-the-job training, reviewing productivity reports, writing job descriptions, scheduling employees, developing policies and procedures, designing performance standards, and developing and implementing goals and objectives for the department. The clinical nutrition manager is also responsible for communicating with the staff of other departments and the administration. Ultimately, the clinical nutrition manager ensures that performance is actually accomplished to achieve the goals and objectives for the department. The Clinical Nutrition Management Dietetic Practice Group provides an excellent yearly workshop on practice updates and opportunities for networking with peers.

Clinical Dietitian

The primary responsibility of the clinical dietitian is to provide nutritional care for patients. Clinical dietitians in hospitals are involved in nutritional screening for patients to determine the presence of or risk of developing malnutrition, to perform nutritional assessments, and to develop nutrition care plans. Clinical nutrition services may be provided to general patient-care units or may be based on a medical specialization (e.g., critical care or diabetes education). Clinical dietitians are important members of the healthcare team because they consult and collaborate with physicians, pharmacists, nurses, social workers, chaplains, and others when providing nutritional care.

Clinical dietitians are the source of authoritative knowledge about MNT and patient nutrition education. They routinely communicate with other disciplines regarding developments in MNT and patient education through in-service teams, rounds, and multidisciplinary patient care conferences.

Successful clinical dietitians in acute healthcare facilities must also be able to apply managerial concepts to provide effective nutritional care. Management tasks often performed by clinical dietitians include scheduling of patient care services, in-service training, on-the-job training, employee interviews and evaluations, writing job descriptions, planning cycle menus, and evaluating the quality of patient food.

Clinical dietitians working in settings other than acute healthcare facilities tend to be involved in a wider range of tasks. Their responsibilities often include more managerial and administrative tasks similar to the duties of a clinical manager. In addition, they may provide more preventive nutrition therapy through instruction on modification of lifestyle.

Typical responsibilities of three different levels of clinical dietitians in a large, acute care hospital are shown in Table 6-3, with an indication of the knowledge, skill, and experience required of each in Table 6-4.

Clinical dietitians may be members of one or more dietetic practice group. Besides working in general clinical practice, dietitians may be gerontological nutritionists, dietitians in developmental and psychiatric disorders, oncology dietitians, renal dietitians, pediatric dietitians, diabetes care and support, dietitians in nutrition support, perinatal nutritionist, and others. The diversity of specialty and subspecialty areas of practice reflects the broad range of interests and opportunities open to the clinical dietitian.

Dietetic Technicians

The dietetic technician in the clinical setting assists the clinical dietitian and is a valuable member of the nutrition care team. At present, there is a

Table 6-3. Clinical Dietitian Responsibilities

Function	Staff	Senior	Specialist
Nutritional screening	X	X	X
Nutritional assessments/care plans:			
Diet instructions	X	X	X
General patients	X	X	X
Critical care/complex patients		X	X
Diet calculations, eating plans, menu checking, evaluation of meal service	X	X	X
Evaluates nutrient intake and provides follow-up care	X	X	X
Directs activities of dietetic technicians and dietetic assistants	X	X	X
Provides clinical in-services to dietitians, dietetic technicians, and dietitian assistants	X	X	X
Participates in performance evaluation of dietetic technicians and dietetic assistants	X	X	X
Medical team rounds and multidisciplinary team meetings	X	X	X
Evaluation of clinical monitors for quality management	X	X	X
On-call duties (weekend/week night)	X	X	X
Clinical nutrition committee membership	X	X	X
Clinical responsibility in focus area— patient education or assessment		X	X
Maintains reference in area of clinical focus		X	X
Revises standards of care and clinical procedures		X	X
Conducts peer review of clinical dietitian chart notes		X	X
Trains new staff interns		X	X

(continues)

Table 6-3. Clinical Dietitian Responsibilities *(continued)*

Function	Staff	Senior	Specialist
Clinical responsibility in area of specialization			X
Provides updates in specialization area			X
Participates in research and presents findings			X
Scheduling dietitian coverage in absence of supervisor			X
Chairs clinical committees		co-chairs	co-chairs

Source: Courtesy of The Methodist Hospital, Houston, Texas, 1998.

shortage of dietetic technicians due to the limited number of educational programs and a growing demand for their services to extend and complement the services of dietitians. Typically, the major functions performed are gathering data for nutritional screening and assigning a level of risk for malnutrition according to predetermined criteria. They may help with nutritional assessments by gathering laboratory and anthropometric data, collecting and analyzing nutritional intake information, obtaining nutritional histories, and reviewing medical histories. Dietetic technicians may administer nourishment and dietary supplements for patients and monitor patient tolerance. They may provide information to help patients select

Table 6-4. Knowledge, Skill, and Experience Requirements for Clinical Dietitians

Function	Staff	Senior	Specialist
Registered Dietitian (the ADA)	Yes	Yes	Yes
Licensure	Yes	Yes	Yes
Clinical experience (years)	Entry	3	5
Advanced knowledge and certification	No	No	Yes
Outside continuing education hours	No	Yes	Yes

Source: Courtesy of The Methodist Hospital, Houston, Texas, 1998.

menus and give simple diet instructions. Dietetic technicians maintain a high level of knowledge of nutritional care. Management responsibilities of dietetic technicians may include supervision of dietetic assistants.

Dietetic Assistants

The dietetic assistant helps the clinical dietitian and dietetic technician in some of the more routine aspects of nutritional care. They are often responsible for processing diet orders, checking menus against standards, setting up standard nourishments, and tallying special food requests. Dietetic assistants may also help distribute and pick up inpatient menus and pass and collect trays. They may be involved in evaluating patient food satisfaction and gathering food records to be used to evaluate nutrient intake.

CLINICAL DIETETICS OUTLOOK

Healthcare Reform

Changes in health care are occurring rapidly. Various bills have been introduced in Congress over time aimed toward reforms of the healthcare system, especially toward providing affordable health care for everyone.[15] The ADA has vigorously lobbied for the inclusion of nutrition care through expansion of MNT at every opportunity and continues to do so. The role of the clinical dietitian will also expand as disease conditions beyond diabetes and renal disease are allowed for reimbursement of services rendered by the RD, such as cardiovascular, obesity, and other diseases.

Realizing that the healthcare debate has great importance to dietitians, the ADA appointed a Health Care Reform Task Group in 2008 to develop association recommendations on healthcare reform.[16] Five major policy positions are recommended by the group as follows:

1. The primary focus of any healthcare initiative must be to improve the health status of Americans. The vital and unique role that nutrition plays in improving and maintaining an individual's health as well as the health of all Americans should be explicit in U.S. health policy.
2. Every American has a fundamental right to the best quality of health care available. This includes access to healthy food and qualified health professionals, such as Registered Dietitians.

3. Nutrition services are critical to comprehensive healthcare delivery systems. Health maintenance, wellness, disease prevention and early detection, delay in disease progression, and intervention in chronic care management are necessary in a comprehensive health policy.
4. The nation has to address the increased costs of health care and act to expand coverage of nutrition services to improve health outcomes, improve the coordination of health care and disease management to include nutrition care provided by the RD in team-based programs and cover preventive and international nutrition services by RD providers.
5. Nutrition education, nutrition assessment, nutrition counseling, and nutrition intervention are examples of the unique knowledge, training, and skills RDs possess.

Public Opinion Survey

In 2008, a nationwide consumer opinion survey of 783 respondents revealed knowledge and attitudes by consumers regarding nutrition and identified trends that have evolved through periodic surveys.[17] Regarding attitudes toward achieving a healthy, nutritious diet, more respondents (43 percent) say they are doing the right things to achieve this while 38 percent say they know they should but aren't. Two-thirds of respondents considered diet and nutrition "very important." The majority were satisfied with the way they eat, but many indicated "it takes too much time to keep track of my diet" or "I need more practical tips to help me eat right." Some 40 percent indicated they did not know or understand guidelines for diet and nutrition. While the trends show some improvement over time, the implications are that dietitians have an important role to play in helping people attain good food and nutrition habits.

Newer Communication Methods

As health care continues to expand beyond the traditional hospital and doctor's office settings, newer methods to reach the public are also being explored. "Telemedicine" and "telehealth" are methods already being used via two-way or one-way television to transmit medical information. Programs by distance may be interactive, offering information exchange, or non-interactive, where information is transmitted but the recipients do not respond. Dietitians increasingly may be participants in such programs to transmit nutrition information in disease conditions. Busey[18] points out both opportunities and pitfalls in such programs that may impact dietitians as they participate. Electronic charting is another process that more hospitals are turning to and this means that the clinical dietitian will need to become knowledgeable about this procedure and be prepared to fully implement it in his or her practice.

Clinical Privileging

Clinical privileging refers to a process by which a hospital, specifically the governing body and the medical staff of the hospital, develop and implement procedures to ensure safe and quality patient care.[19,20] In most hospitals, the physician is the person responsible for overall patient care and assumes the risk and legal responsibility for the care, including prescribing specific diet orders. The dietetics profession has long discussed the possibility of the dietitian writing the diet order and ordering certain tests based on his or her certification, training, and experience.[21] Referred to as "prescriptive authority," this can only occur if the RD can demonstrate competence in advanced-level skills, is licensed by the state, and has specifically been approved by the hospital. To be considered, the RD must understand that certain legal responsibilities are assumed and that adherence to the Scope of Dietetic Practice is a personal responsibility that will be periodically reviewed by the hospital and the medical staff.[22] Both federal and state regulations apply in the process of clinical privileging; however, as clinical dietitians attain advanced-level training and demonstrate competence and ability, it is likely that more dietitians will assume this responsibility in the future.

A study in 2008 that included 1500 clinical nutrition managers, looked at the prescriptive authority and barriers to such authority of RDs in acute healthcare facilities.[23] Fifty-four percent reported no prescriptive authority, 36% reported dependent authority, and 10% reported independent authority. Dependent authority refers to RDs being able to order diets, nutritional supplements, nutrition-related tests according to pre-approved criteria while independent authority means the RD may perform these tasks with more autonomy.

SUMMARY

The future roles of clinical dietitians will expand as new skills and competencies through advanced training and education are attained. Employment opportunities will include community-based programs, consultation and private practice, communications, and a broad range of entrepreneurial possibilities.

The clinical dietitian is central in helping persons during illness through nutrition interventions. Equally important is helping individuals prevent the onset of chronic disease by the application of optimal nutrition practices throughout life. The expansion of MNT with cost-effectiveness data and demonstration of quality practice is a continuing challenge for the dietetics profession. Even though employment increasingly moves outside the traditional hospital or clinic, the services provided by the clinical dietitian will remain vital to the health and well-being of people experiencing illness and who need nutritional care.

DEFINITIONS

Clinical Dietetics. The area of practice in which persons with illness or injury are treated by using nutrition assessment, planning, and implementation of nutrition care plans.

Clinical Nutrition Services. Activities provided in the practice of clinical dietetics, such as medical nutrition therapy and counseling.

Diet Therapy. Treatment by diet; this term is now replaced by "clinical nutrition therapy" or "medical nutrition therapy."

Extended Care Facility. An institution that extends health care beyond the acute care setting; when long-term care is needed.

Medical Nutrition Therapy. The application of nutrition in the management of illness or injury.

Outpatient Clinic. Treatment area of a hospital or healthcare facility in which patients are treated on an outpatient basis.

REFERENCES

1. Coulston, A.M. and C.L. Rock. "A Summary of the Current State of Knowledge in Clinical Nutrition and Dietetic Practice: Suggestions for Future Research in Dietetic Practice and Implications for Health Care." In *The Research Agenda for Dietitians.* ADA Conference Proceedings. The American Dietetic Association: Chicago; 1993, pp. 1–24.
2. Cooper, L.F. "The Dietitian and Her Profession." *J Am Diet Assoc* 14(1938): 751–758.
3. Huyck, L. and M.M. Rowe. *Managing Clinical Nutrition Services.* Aspen Publishers: Rockville, MD; 1990, p. 243.

4. Butterworth, E. "The Skeleton in the Hospital Closet." *Nutrition Today* 9(1974): 4.
5. American Dietetic Association. Compensation and Benefits Survey of the Dietetic Profession 2009. www.eatright.org. Accessed October 20, 2009.
6. Lacey, K. and E. Pritchett. "Nutrition Care Process and Model: ADA Adopts Road Map to Quality Care and Outcomes Management." *J Am Diet Assoc* 103, no. 8(2003): 1061–1071.
7. Ibid.
8. Writing Group of the Nutrition Care Process and Standardized Language Committee. "Nutrition Care Process and Model Part I: The 2008 Update. *J Am Diet Assoc* 108, no. 7(2008): 1113–1117.
9. Writing Group of the Nutrition Care Process and Standardized Language Committee. "Nutrition Care Process and Model Part II: Using the International Dietetics and Nutrition Terminology to Document the Nutrition Care Process." *J Am Diet Assoc* 108, no. 8(2008): 1287–1293.
10. Smith, R.E., S. Patrick., P. Michael, and M. Hager. "Medical Nutrition Therapy: The Case of ADA's Advocacy Efforts (Part I)." *J Am Diet Assoc* 105, no. 5(2005): 825–834.
11. Smith, R.E., S. Patrick, P. Michael, and M. Hager. "Medical Nutrition Therapy: The Case of ADA's Advocacy Efforts. (Part II)." *J Am Diet Assoc* 105, no. 6(2005): 987–996.
12. Ibid.
13. Blumberg-Kason, S. and R. Lipscomb. "Evidence-Based Nutrition Practice Guidelines: A Valuable Resource in the Evidence-Analysis Library." *J Am Diet Assoc* 106, no. 12(2006): 1935–1936.
14. ADA. "2008 Standards of Practice in Nutrition Care for RDs and DTRs." www.eatright.org (Accessed April 10, 2009).
15. See Note 10.
16. ADA. "Health Care Reform." December 2008. www.eatright.org (Accessed April 20, 2009).
17. ADA. "Nutrition and You: Trends 2008." www.eatright.org (Accessed April 25, 2009).
18. Busey, J.C. and P. Michael. "Telehealth—Opportunities and Pitfalls." *J Am Diet Assoc* 108, no. 8(2008): 1296–1301.
19. Hager, M.H. "Clinical Privileging for Registered Dietitians. A Regulatory Perspective." *J Am Diet Assoc* 107, no. 4(2007): 558–560.
20. Hager, M.H. and S.M. McCauley. "Clinical Privileging: What It Is . . . And Isn't." *J Am Diet Assoc* 109, no. 3(2009): 400–402.
21. See Note 19.
22. See Note 20.
23. Weil, S.D., L. Lafferty, K.S. Keim, D. Sowa, and R. Dowling. "Registered Dietitian Prescriptive Practices in Hospitals." *J Am Diet Assoc* 108, no. 10(2008): 1688–1692.

CHAPTER 7

Management in Food and Nutrition Systems

"Knowledge of food and management skills is essential to most areas of practice in dietetics. Many dietetic practice groups, including those in clinical nutrition, community nutrition and business practice, routinely translate nutrition science into food choices for specific audiences."[1]

OUTLINE

- Introduction
- Areas of Employment
  - Food and Nutrition Management in Acute Care
  - Food and Nutrition Management in Long-Term Care
  - Food and Nutrition Management in Noninstitutional Settings
  - School Nutrition Programs
  - Clinical Nutrition Management
  - Commercial Food Services
  - Further Areas of Opportunity
- Standards for Professional Performance
  - Characteristics of Successful Food and Nutrition Managers
- Expanded Opportunities
- Summary

INTRODUCTION

Food and food service are prominent in the history of the profession of dietetics. One of the main purposes of the first organized meeting of the American Dietetic Association was to discuss ways of meeting food shortages during World War I. Many of the first members of the association served overseas feeding hospitalized soldiers and people living under wartime conditions. Cooking schools, scientists who produced the first tables of food values, early day soup kitchens, and school lunch programs were among the forerunners of institutions that fed the public.[2]

Food service in hospitals was the primary focus of the first dietitians. During the 1890s, food service in hospitals was managed by the chef, the housekeeper, or the nursing department. In the early 1900s, however, many dietitians were in charge of dietary departments and had the responsibility for all food service as well as teaching nurses and providing diet therapy for patients with metabolic diseases. Hospital dietitians dealt with budgets, department organization, personnel management, and quality food service. Nutrition was recognized as an aspect of medicine, and food prescriptions were handled as apothecary compounds, thus creating a demand for special diet kitchens. The hospital dietitian had the same status as the superintendent of nurses and was recognized as the nutrition expert.[3]

Dietitians with food service management responsibilities became members of the Food Administration section in the ADA and their practice was referred to as "administrative dietetics." The terminology now used is "management in food and nutrition systems."

Spears[4] defines the manager as "one who is responsible for people and organizational resources and possesses management skills including technical, human, and conceptual." In this chapter, the focus is on the dietitian in food service and management and the manager in clinical services.

AREAS OF EMPLOYMENT

The majority of dietitians begin their career in clinical practice. In 2009, however, 21 percent of those participating in the compensation and benefits study indicated they were dietitians or managers and another 15 percent were supervisors or coordinators.[5] The results are similar for RDs and DTRs. Forty three percent of RDs and 47 percent of DTRs directly or indirectly supervise employees. Twenty-five percent of RDs and 23 percent of

DTRs manage a budget. The findings are a strong indicator that more than half of practicing dietitians and DTRs are performing managerial functions.

In the same 2009 study, it was reported that salaries for the food and nutrition manager are among the highest of those in any practice area, second only to those in consultation and business. The salaries reflect both geographic location as well as years of experience as the food and nutrition manager is usually a dietitian with work experience beyond entry level and may have an advanced degree or a business degree.

Dietitians in food and nutrition management typically affiliate with four ADA dietetic practice groups: Management in Food and Nutrition Systems, Dietitians in Business and Communication, School Nutrition Services, and Food and Culinary Professionals. In addition, clinical managers may belong to the Clinical Nutrition Management Group. Dietitians in food and nutrition management may be identified through a wide range of titles. For instance, titles of coordinator, specialist, and executive dietitian are used. Among traditional titles, Liu[6] further found position titles of director or associate director of food and nutrition services, director of clinical nutrition, director of multi-unit services, and food and nutrition consultant. Molt[7] described titles such as director, chief, or chief administrator among dietitians working in hospital food service, school food service, and college and university residence halls.

Practice areas are often categorized by work settings, such as food and nutrition management in acute care, long-term care, and noninstitutional employment areas. To encompass the broader management area, clinical nutrition management, commercial food service, and school nutrition are added to this list. A brief discussion of each of these follows.

Food and Nutrition Management in Acute Care

Food service in acute care is the type of service provided in hospitals or similar healthcare institutions in which patients receive short-term medical treatment, usually 1 to 5 days. Several characteristics of this type of food service are:

1. fast turnover of patients with day-to-day fluctuations in the number of meals prepared and served
2. special diets requiring different types of food preparation. In some instances, as many as 30 to 50 percent of all patients will require special or modified diets.

3. selective menus for patients, increasing the number of food items prepared
4. multiple serving systems in an institution, such as individual tray service for patients, cafeteria service and vending for hospital personnel and the public, and catering for hospital staff
5. various types of food service such as centralized tray service, decentralized service with pantries on patient floors, and restaurant-style service providing individualized patient service

In some institutions, food is prepared in bulk then pre-portioned and held until the time of meal service when it is rethermalized and served. In others, food is prepared centrally just before meal service and either portioned individually or sent in bulk to patient areas for individual service. Production and service systems vary but in each system, the dietitian has overall responsibility for food production and service or may share this responsibility with a chef or a manager. Whatever the scope of his or her responsibility, the dietitian must be knowledgeable in food production techniques, food purchasing, safety and sanitation, strategic planning, human relations, communication skill, managerial skills, and financial management.

Food and Nutrition Management in Long-Term Care

The provision of food for clients in nursing homes, extended care facilities, and correctional institutions is included in this category. Food service in these institutions differs from that in acute care in that clients are long term and are usually served in group settings. Central food production and few special diets are typical because most of the long-term clients will be following a normal, healthy eating pattern. The food service, especially in smaller nursing homes and extended care facilities, may be managed by a dietetic technician or by a certified dietary manager under the direction of a dietitian consultant. In correctional institutions, the day-to-day management is often provided by nonprofessionals under the direction of a dietitian consultant when one is available. All aspects of food service management are equally as important in long-term care as in the hospital, with the added necessity of ensuring nutritional adequacy and acceptability over longer periods of time. There are federal and state regulations relating to the provision of food services to clients in almost all long-term facilities that must be followed for the institution to receive funding and provide quality care. The qualifications for the food service manager are also specified in the regulations.

Food and Nutrition Management in Noninstitutional Settings

This type of management is typically provided in colleges and universities, employee cafeterias, and business and commercial enterprises. The food service may be for-profit or nonprofit, depending on the type of institution. Generally, institutions serving the public will be for-profit while schools or businesses providing employee food services generally will be nonprofit. Clients choose to patronize the food services offered and the types of food services may vary widely. A college or university, for instance, may offer cafeteria, dining room, restaurant, catering, and vending services. School and employee food service is often provided by cafeteria service along with vending and dining room service. Many businesses provide employee cafeterias or restaurant service. The dietitian's responsibility is to provide food that is safe and acceptable to the customers, meets financial expectations, and promotes good nutrition.

School Nutrition Programs

School nutrition programs, offering either lunch or breakfast, or both, are available in 99 percent of all public schools and 83 percent of all public and private schools combined.[8] In 2007, about 31 million students from preschool to grade 12 were fed daily.[8] An average of 10 million children per day participated in the school breakfast program in 2007. The programs are administered and partially funded by the federal government and they must meet specific guidelines for nutritional quality of meals and for student eligibility. Free meals are provided based on the family economic status. The emphasis is on long-term health benefits for children through establishing good eating habits. The following is a position statement supporting school nutrition programs:

> It is the position of the American Dietetic Association, the Society for Nutrition Education, and the American School Food Service Association [now the School Nutrition Association] that comprehensive nutrition services must be provided to all of the nation's preschool through grade twelve students. These nutrition services shall be integrated with a coordinated, comprehensive school health program and implemented through a school nutrition policy. The policy should link comprehensive sequential nutrition education; access to and promotion of child

nutrition programs providing nutritious meals and snacks in the school environment; and family, community, and health services' partnerships supporting positive health outcomes for all children.[9]

Dietitians in school nutrition programs need both managerial and nutrition education skills. Many in this career area affiliate with the School Nutrition Services DPG and also the School Nutrition Association.

The National Food Service Management Institute conducts research regarding the functions and tasks of school nutrition managers. The job functions rated most important are program accountability, sanitation and safety, customer service, equipment use and care, and food production. The manager in a school nutrition program has responsibilities in at least seven other areas: nutrition and menu planning, food procurement, food acceptability, financial management, marketing, personnel management, and professional development.[10]

Clinical Nutrition Management

Clinical nutrition management refers to the activities of practitioners in hospitals and healthcare institutions who develop and operate systems that successfully meet the nutritional needs of patients.[11] This may include the responsibility for one or more units and the supervision of other professionals in clinical areas. The clinical manager performs many of the same management functions as the food service dietitian: management of human, financial, and material resources. The clinical dietitian who progresses from an entry-level position to a management position will normally have 5 to 10 years or more of experience and will not be involved in day-to-day activities directly related to patient care.

Commercial Food Services

Commercial food service is described as retail and hospitality food service establishments that prepare food for immediate consumption on or off premises. The types of establishments employing dietitians include independent restaurants, casual and family dining restaurants, and fine dining restaurants. Supermarket chains, limited service (fast-food) chains, and hotel chains also have high potential for dietetic services. Five specific areas of need in these institutions are: nutrition education, healthful menu planning, recipe and menu analysis, marketing, and quality assurance.

Skills in public relations, communications, marketing, purchasing, and financial management are expected of dietitians who work in commercial food services. Therefore, additional training and experience are often needed by the dietitian to be fully qualified for these roles.

Further Areas of Opportunity

Further opportunities for dietitians in food service management include positions in food corporations, such as research and development, consumer affairs, communications, government liaison; disaster planning centers; military bases; homeless shelters and food distribution centers; worldwide religious ministries and government food programs; and academic units with food, nutrition, or hospitality programs. Many dietitians are employed in contract food service companies that provide for-profit management services. Hospitals, colleges and universities, schools, employee cafeterias in businesses, hotels and restaurants, and healthcare institutions may contract with a company who manages food services for a negotiated fee. The companies hire and often train their own personnel including dietitian managers.

STANDARDS FOR PROFESSIONAL PERFORMANCE

Several studies, important to ADA members, have been conducted to determine what the dietitian in various areas of practice is expected to accomplish in the performance of the job. A 1996 study pointed to the percentage of time spent by dietitians in food and nutrition management at the entry level and beyond.[12] The study indicated that experienced dietitians spent more time in advising, policy setting, and supervising, while the less experienced and entry-level dietitians were more involved in carrying out day-to-day activities. The experienced dietitian also participated in a broader range of activities, including teaching, research, and marketing.

In 2000, an ADA group developed standards for professional practice in management and food service—a first innovative step.[13] The standards described the minimum expectations in management and food service settings for the quality of service, the analysis of practices performed, and the services that maximize the nutritional health and well-being of clients or customers. The standards applied to the following areas of practice: application of research, communication, application of knowledge, utilization and management of resources, and quality in practice. The standards included the rationale, indicators, and examples of outcomes.

In 2005, Standards of Practice (SOP) and Standards of Professional Performance (SOPP) were developed by the association for nutrition care.[14] The standards were updated in 2008.[15] These are general standards in that they outline activities that apply in all areas of dietetics practice. They have become the blueprint for the development of standards in all areas of practice.

The general standards provide for the following activities:

- describe minimum levels of practice and performance
- provide common indicators for self-evaluation
- promote consistency in practice and performance
- describe the role of dietetics and the unique services that RDs and DTRs provide within the healthcare team
- illustrate that food and nutrition services are provided in a framework that encourages continuous quality improvement
- provide a basis for researchers to investigate relationships between dietetics practice and outcomes
- provide a framework for educators to set objectives for educational programs
- reflect applicable federal laws and regulations

The management standards that build on the 2005 and 2008 general standards are statements that describe a competent level of professionalism and the professional role behaviors that relate to quality of care and administrative practice, resource management, education, professional environment, ethics, collaboration, research, and resource allocation.[16] According to Puckett,[17] today's management RD must, at a minimum, possess competencies in the following areas:

- environmental protection rules
- the political environment
- marketing and customer satisfaction
- continual quality improvement
- work design and productivity
- innovative cost-containment measures
- food consumption patterns
- human resources trends
- food and water safety
- disaster and emergency planning

- project and process management
- cultural diversity in the marketplace

Characteristics of Successful Food and Nutrition Managers

Dietitians in food and nutrition management need to exhibit leadership qualities similar to those in all areas of business, healthcare institutions, schools, and the like. They must manage personnel and financial resources, produce quality products and services, and communicate effectively within the organization and to the larger community. The development of "transformational leaders," defined as those who possess personal characteristics that allow them to influence the work situation, was studied by Arensberg and colleagues.[18] The transformational leader helps people and organizations function at a high level, to master change, and to plan futuristically.

A list of leadership competencies needed by healthcare food service directors is shown in Table 7-1. The competencies are typical of visionary leaders who are effective in their positions and in the organization.

Table 7-1. Leadership Competencies Needed by Healthcare Food Service Directors

Successful healthcare food service directors will:

- Exhibit astute collaborative management techniques to unify diverse points of view through consensus building, to cultivate mutually advantageous relationships in and out of the institution, and to achieve cooperation through teamwork.
- Demonstrate effective communication techniques to achieve a common understanding of personnel and departmental policies, and effective interpersonal skills through two-way communication with personnel inside and outside the department.
- Achieve an organizational structure, mission statement, policies, and procedures that effect necessary changes while managing risk-taking for the department.
- Possess common-sense intelligence based on sound technological knowledge of food service, practice experience, and consideration of external business and administrative needs.
- Bear effective personnel management techniques based on sound character, compassion, insight, and personal integrity.
- Exhibit personal behaviors and attitudes consistent with professional and institutional goals.

(continues)

Table 7-1. Leadership Competencies Needed by Healthcare Food Service Directors *(continued)*

- Demonstrate continuing pursuit of professional knowledge and growth.
- Possess effective supervisory and managerial techniques to derive optimal employee performance and appropriate documentation.
- Achieve ways to enhance performance and growth of employees.
- Possess an understanding of the politics of the institution and an ability to interface effectively with superiors.
- Exhibit effective use of resources (e.g., fiscal, personnel, materials) to facilitate planning and current operations.
- Possess analytic and decision-making techniques to achieve maximum quality for customers and clients.
- Personify behaviors and techniques that foster professional growth and leadership in department personnel.
- Demonstrate the ability to formulate a creative vision for the department that integrates mutually satisfying department and institutional goals.

Source: Watabe-Dawson, M. "Visionary Leaders Are Key to Success in Food Service." Copyright The American Dietetic Association. Reprinted by permission from *Journal of the American Dietetic Association,* vol. 95, p. 13, © 1995.

EXPANDED OPPORTUNITIES

Entry-level dietitians with management responsibilities are employed primarily in food service or clinical nutrition service operations. The predominant responsibilities at this level involve technical skills that ensure that food is procured, managed, prepared, and delivered to patients and other clients, and that appropriate nutrition services are provided. With experience and perhaps advanced study, conceptual skills are utilized to identify problem areas requiring attention, to select appropriate techniques, to analyze alternative strategies, and to select solutions consistent with organization goals.

From entry-level positions, dietitians may advance to the assistant or associate director level of a department, and eventually to director or chief administrator. They may manage multi-departmental units or a complex of smaller hospitals, specialty clinics, or long-term care centers. They may become the Chief Operating Officer of a healthcare facility.

Dietitians directing food and nutrition services must have a diversified multipurpose, broad-based education and experiences from which to draw for expanded roles. They must be familiar with applicable computer software, business organization, marketing, labor relations, industrial engineering, writing and media relations, public relations, financial management, data evaluation, policy formation and problem solving, decision making, negotiation skill, behavior modification techniques, and dealing with adaptive challenges.[19]

Expanded roles may include new and challenging positions that grow from the foundation the dietitian receives and that may not even generally be associated with dietetics. In health care, for instance, there is heightened consumer interest in what constitutes "healthy" food. The food industry wants effective marketing of their products, including information about the safety and nutrient value, and they want to develop new products. All these areas represent opportunities in consumer education, writing, food safety, media positions, public policy, food demonstrations, and more.

SUMMARY

The dietitian in food service management has career opportunities in foods, food production and service, management, and the higher levels of activities associated with management and leadership. For the motivated and skilled dietitian, higher salary levels and greater degrees of responsibility and self-actualization can be realized.

DEFINITIONS

Food Production. The process of preparing and serving food, including purchasing, storage, and processing.

Food Services. Production and service of food; also refers to the unit or group responsible for feeding groups, usually in an institutional setting.

Food Service Systems. Activities that together form the inputs, transformation, and outputs that make up an entire food operation.

Human Resources. The personnel in an organization.

Management. Administration and coordination of the activities and functions in an organizational unit.

Quality Assurance. Certification of the continual, optimal, effective, and efficient outcomes of a service or program.

Resource Allocation. Equitable distribution of financial, physical, and human capital.

Transformation. Action or activity that changes input into output in a system.

REFERENCES

1. Halling, J.F. and M.A. Hess. "Vision vs. Reality: ADA Members as Food/Food Management Experts." *J Am Diet Assoc* 95(1995): 169–170.
2. Cassell, J.A. *Carry the Flame: The History of the American Dietetic Association.* The American Dietetic Association: Chicago; 1990.
3. Barker, A., M. Foltz, M.B.F. Arensberg, and M.R. Schiller. *Leadership in Dietetics: Achieving a Vision for the Future.* The American Dietetic Association: Chicago; 1994, p. 54.
4. Spears, M.C. *Foodservice Organization: A Managerial and Systems Approach.* 3rd ed. Englewood Cliffs, NJ: Prentice Hall; 1995, p. 202.
5. American Dietetic Association. Compensation and Benefits Survey of the Dietetics Profession 2009. www.eatright.org. Accessed October 15, 2009.
6. Liu, Y.A. "Incentives Perceived by Management Dietitians to Reduce Absenteeism Rate of Foodservice Personnel in Health Care Systems." Stillwater, Oklahoma; 1996. Unpublished PhD dissertation.
7. Molt, M.K. "Dietitian's Ratings of Helpfulness of Experiences to Their Leadership Development." *Journal of the National Association of College & University Food Services* 19(1995): 41–50.
8. Story, M. "The Third School Nutrition Dietary Assessment Study: Findings and Policy Implications for Improving the Health of U.S. Citizens." *J Am Diet Assoc* 109, no. 2(2009): S7–13.
9. Briggs, M., S. Safaii, D.L. Beall, American Dietetic Association, Society for Nutrition Education, and American School Food Service Association. "Position of the American Dietetic Association, Society for Nutrition Education and American School Food Service Association—Nutrition Services: An Essential Component of Comprehensive School Health Programs." *J Am Diet Assoc* 103, no. 4(2003): 505–514.
10. National Food Service Management Institute. "Job Functions and Tasks of School Nutrition Managers and District Managers/Supervisors." University of Mississippi-Oxford; 1995, p. 5.
11. Jackson, R. *Nutrition and Food Services for Integrated Health Care.* Aspen Publishers: Gaithersburg, MD; 1997, p. 170.
12. Kane, M.T., A.S. Estes, D.A. Colton, and C.S. Eltoft. "Commission on Dietetic Registration Dietetics Practice Audit." *J Am Diet Assoc* 96(1996): 1124–1133.

13. Griffin B., J.M. Dunn, J. Irwin, and I.F. Speranza. "Standards of Professional Practice for Dietetics Professionals in Management and Food Service Settings." *J Am Diet Assoc* 101, no. 8(2001): 944–946.
14. Kieselhorst, K., J. Skates, and E. Pritchett. "American Dietetic Association: Standards of Practice in Nutrition Care and Updated Standards of Professional Performance." *J Am Diet Assoc* 105(2005): 641–645.
15. American Dietetic Association Quality Management Committee. "American Dietetic Association Revised 2008 Standards of Practice for Registered Dietitians in Nutrition Care; Standards of Professional Performance for Registered Dietitians; Standards of Practice for Dietetic Technicians, Registered, in Nutrition Care; and Standards of Professional Performance for Dietetic Technicians, Registered." *J Am Diet Assoc* 108, no. 9(2008): 1538–1542.
16. Puckett, R.P., W. Barkley, G. Dixon, K. Egan, C. Koch, T. Malone, J. Scott-Smith, B. Sheridan, and M. Theis. "The American Dietetic Association Standards of Professional Performance for Registered Dietitians (Generalist and Advanced) in Management of Food and Nutrition Systems." *J Am Diet Assoc* 109, no. 3(2009): 540–543.
17. Puckett, R. "Leadership: Managing for Change." In *Food Service Manual for Health Care Institutions.* 3rd ed. Jossey-Bass: San Francisco, CA; 2004, pp. 30–32.
18. Arensberg, M.B.F., M.R. Schiller, V.N. Vivian, W.A. Johnson, and S. Strasser. "Transformational Leadership of Clinical Nutrition Managers." *J Am Diet Assoc* 96(1996): 39–45.
19. Heifetz, R.A. and D.Z. Laurie. "The Work of Leadership." *Harvard Bus Rev* 75(1997): 124–134.

The Community Nutrition Dietitian

"Primary prevention is the most effective and affordable course of action for preventing and reducing the risk for chronic disease."[1]

OUTLINE

- Introduction
- Community Nutrition Practice
- Public Health Nutrition
  - Prevention
  - Levels of Prevention
- Activities of Community Dietitians
- Career Paths
  - Specialty Areas of Practice
- Career Outlook
- Summary

INTRODUCTION

Community nutrition is the branch of nutrition that addresses the entire range of food and nutrition issues relating to individuals, families, and special groups with a common bond such as place of residence, language, culture, and health. Community nutrition programs include those that

117

provide increased access to food resources, food and nutrition education, and health care. Public health nutrition is the component of community nutrition that is publicly funded and provided through a state or local health agency to promote health, prevent disease, and provide primary care. The community dietitian, community nutritionist, or public health nutritionist is the dietetic professional who provides nutrition services to identified groups.

Community nutrition professionals establish links with other professionals involved with the broad range of human services, including child-care agencies, services to the elderly, educational institutions, and community-based research. They focus on promoting optimum health and preventing disease in the community by using a population and systems focus and a client or personal health service approach.[2]

COMMUNITY NUTRITION PRACTICE

Community and public health dietitians work in many settings that focus on improving the health of a population group. Positions are characterized by an emphasis on health and wellness and the application of nutrition science to maintain health. Community dietitians often work in federal, state, or local public health agencies; neighborhood or community health centers; industry; ambulatory care clinics; home health agencies and specialized community projects; nonprofit and for-profit private and community health agencies; institutions; private practice; and hospitals.

Each state has a department of health employing public health dietitians. Many states also use dietitians or nutritionists in programs such as Native American health service, health and human services or welfare, department of education (school nutrition programs), and in area agencies for the aging. The land-grant university in each state administers the cooperative extension program in which nutritionists, nutrition educators, and expanded food and nutrition educators are employed.

PUBLIC HEALTH NUTRITION

Practice in community nutrition is characterized by a focus on the community and includes those activities that are focused on groups rather than individuals. The largest sub-unit of community nutrition is public health nutrition. Whereas the practice area of community nutrition tends to be large and has a small body of defining literature, public health nutrition is well defined and includes a large body of literature discussing its role and defining characteristics. Public health dietitians or nutritionists tend to work in federal, state, or local agencies.

To understand what a public health dietitian does requires familiarity with the field of public health. The public health population-based or epidemiologic approach is distinguished from the clinical or one-on-one care approach.[3] Public health focuses on the society as a whole, and the community, for the provision of optimal health. The mission of public health is the fulfillment of society's interest in ensuring the conditions in which individuals can be healthy.[4] The goal of the discipline is to promote optimal nutrition and health for all members of the population by improving nutritional status and maintaining health.[5]

A leading public health nutritionist defines a public health nutritionist as "the member of the public health agency staff who is responsible for planning, organizing, managing, directing, coordinating and evaluating the nutrition component of the health agency's services. The public health nutritionist establishes linkages with related community nutrition programs, nutrition education, food assistance, social or welfare services, care services to the elderly, other human services and community-based research."[6]

The public health approach has the following characteristics:

- Uses interventions that promote health and prevent communicable or chronic diseases by managing or controlling the community environment
- Promotes a healthy lifestyle as a shared value for all people
- Directs money and energy to the problems that affect the lives of the largest number of people in the community
- Targets the unserved or underserved by virtue of income, age, ethnicity, heredity, or lifestyle who are vulnerable to disease, hunger, or malnutrition
- Requires the collaboration of the public, consumers, community leaders, legislators, policy makers, administrators, and health and human service professionals in assessing and responding to community needs and consumer demands
- Monitors the health of the people in the community to ensure that the public health system achieves its objectives and responds to needs

Prevention

The prevention of illness is the primary purpose of public health. Prevention may take place at any point along the spectrum from prevention of disease to the prevention of impairment or disability. Prevention has three essential components:

1. personal health
2. community-based
3. social policies or systems-based

Each component has distinct roles, importance, and focus. Community nutrition practice involves making appropriate and coordinated use of each. Personal health deals with prevention issues at the individual level, such as working with a client to improve the diet for health promotion purposes. Community-based prevention uses campaigns that focus, for example, on increased consumption of fruits and vegetables or weight maintenance. Social policies or systems-level prevention focuses on changing policies and law so that the goals of prevention practice are achieved, such as laws regarding food safety, tobacco, or alcohol.

Levels of Prevention

For each of the three components of prevention, there are three levels of prevention. Primary prevention or health promotion efforts involve prevention of the disease itself and serve to maintain a state of wellness. Secondary prevention is the detection, diagnosis, and intervention early in the disease process to minimize disabling effects. Tertiary prevention is directed at treating and rehabilitating persons with diagnosed health conditions to prevent or delay their disability, pain, suffering, and premature death.[7]

ACTIVITIES OF COMMUNITY DIETITIANS

About 11 percent of RDs and 10 percent of DTRs work in community nutrition.[8] The Women, Infants, and Children Program (WIC) employs 5 percent of the RDs and 8 percent of the DTRs. WIC provides food and nutrition education and works to provide access to health services for low-income pregnant, breastfeeding, and nonbreastfeeding women and their children up to 5 years of age. Other positions include maternal and child nutrition, adult health, food service management, and children with special healthcare needs.

For individuals to benefit from nutrition research, dietitians working in the community must be able to translate science into practical dietary guidance. In useful terms, this means providing information about foods that are affordable and available in local markets. All dietitians must be experts in normal and clinical nutrition and be competent in bringing about changes in eating behavior. To be a credible nutrition resource, the RD who works in the community must understand the fundamentals of nutrition, food science, and dietetics, as well as have an underlying knowledge of human physiology, chemistry, biochemistry, and behavioral sciences. This includes an in-depth knowledge of nutritional needs during all stages of the life span because people of all ages will be served in the various programs.

In practice, dietitians in community programs are knowledgeable in and possess skills in several critical areas. These include:[9]

- Assesses and prioritizes nutrition problems for various age and population groups using anthropometric, biochemical, clinical, dietary, and socioeconomic techniques
- Utilizes federal, regional, state, and local governmental structures and processes involved in the development of public policy, legislation, and regulations that influence and relate to nutrition and health services
- Understands political and ethical considerations within and across organizations and their impact on agency planning, policy, and decision making
- Integrates nutrition services into the overall health agency mission, goals, and plans
- Knows and uses an epidemiologic approach to assess the health and nutrition problems and trends in the community
- Uses processes of monitoring, technical assistance, guidance, consultation, and collaboration within and across agencies and organizations
- Functions as a multidisciplinary and interdisciplinary team member or leader
- Applies skills in selecting and/or developing nutrition education materials and approaches appropriate for individuals or small groups within the target population
- Uses media strategies in print, broadcasting, and telecommunications, such as video and the Internet, to reach population groups

The dietitian's duties may include training of other agency staff as well as providing technical assistance to other professionals; serving as a resource to the public, media, business, and industry; and advocating for needed nutrition policy at the local, state, and/or federal level. Other responsibilities may include advising the agency administrator, policy makers, and staff on current nutrition research that can contribute to the public's health and to the organization's mission, policies, and programs.

CAREER PATHS

The term public health nutritionist has usually been reserved for the member of the nutrition team who has a master's degree in public health nutrition. This training includes skills required to participate in policy analysis and program development. The public health nutritionist knows the practical aspects of assessing the nutritional needs of a community and develops skills in planning, evaluating, and implementing programs to meet these needs. Academic training includes a knowledge of biostatistics and skill in collecting, compiling, analyzing, and reporting demographic, health, and food consumption data, as well as an understanding of the epidemiology of health and disease distribution patterns in the population and trends over time. According to Dodds and Kaufman,[10] public health nutrition personnel can be placed in three major groups based on their responsibilities: management, professional, or technical. The groups are shown in Table 8-1.

Specialty Areas of Practice

Several career paths are available to the public health nutritionist in areas considered specialties. Typical of these are the following:

Adult health promotion or chronic disease prevention and control specialists may work in healthcare facilities, worksite health promotion, and community health agencies. Knowledge of nutritional management of specific chronic diseases and behavioral and lifestyle change methodologies is required.

Specialists working with special healthcare needs related to developmental diseases and chronic disabling conditions need clinical knowledge of child growth and development with an emphasis on the effects of mental retardation, developmental disabilities, and re-

Table 8-1. Positions of Public Health Nutritionists

Class	Type of Position	Functions
Management	Public Health Director Assistant Public Health Director	Policy making, planning, management, supervision, fiscal control
Professional	Public Health Nutrition Consultant Public Health Nutritionist Clinical Nutritionist Nutritionist	Planning and evaluation, consultation, case management, counseling
Technical	Nutrition Technician Nutrition Assistant	Education, screening, recordkeeping, outreach

Source: Adapted with permission from Dodds, J.M. and M. Kaufman. *Personnel in Public Health Nutrition for the 1990s. A Comprehensive Guide.* Washington, D.C.: The Public Health Foundation; 1991.

habilitation. Knowledge of techniques of feeding under special conditions is also required.

Maternal and child health specialists understand principles of nutrition in pregnancy and lactation and in infancy, childhood, and adolescence. This includes the physical, psychological, and socioeconomic aspects of these early periods of life.

Communication and media specialists must have knowledge of how individuals learn and of nutrition education methodology. They must also know how to use media effectively to design and implement nutrition promotion campaigns through a variety of communication channels, including television, radio, newspapers, magazines, and computers in various settings.

Data management and nutrition surveillance nutritionists require additional training in biostatistics and epidemiology, and computer-based data management. Their responsibilities include the development of user-friendly systems for collecting, analyzing, interpreting, and presenting numerical data to be used in community program planning.

Environmental health and food safety specialists have advanced knowledge and skills in food science, food processing technology, microbiology, epidemiology, and food safety laws and regulations. They must be able to interpret federal, state, and local regulations regarding food safety.

Food service systems management for healthcare and group care facilities specialists have in-depth knowledge of food service systems management, healthcare financing, clinical nutrition, and nutritional care planning.

Home health specialists have advanced knowledge of diet therapy for chronic disease and chronic disabling conditions of adults and children.

Research specialists need to know how to prepare grant proposals, manage data, coordinate field-based studies, and design research protocols.

Educators of public health nutrition professionals must have the knowledge and skills to prepare students for practice in public health or community health.

CAREER OUTLOOK

Community nutrition practice is changing as the overall healthcare system evolves. Expanding opportunities during a time of economic depression require dietitians working in the community to be well prepared academically to compete. At the same time, more nutrition personnel with advanced clinical skills are needed to provide intensive nutritional care in the home and community to medically high-risk pregnant women, disabled and chronically ill infants and children, chronically ill adults, and the elderly.

Public health agencies are expected to assume additional focused responsibilities, and professionals may shift from a client-focused system with direct care responsibilities to a population or system focus with more administrative and planning-related functions. Some in public health will continue to provide personal health services, particularly in areas where providers are limited or where certain high-risk populations are underserved. This shift from a client to a population focus will occur at different rates. In communities where access to clinical, preventive, and therapeutic services are limited, the transition will be slow. Public health and community nutrition professionals will need to be proactive and creative in assuming their responsibilities.

SUMMARY

Community nutrition is an area in which professionals interact with community groups and individuals to promote health and prevent disease. Dietitians and nutritionists working in community nutrition hold positions in areas of public health, programs for the aging, cooperative extension outpatient and public health clinics, state and local governments, and agencies dealing with chronic disease. The emphasis is on meeting the nutritional needs of persons during all stages of life, thus maintaining health and preventing disease.

DEFINITIONS

Client. The recipient of services or products.

Client-Based Focus. Use of assessment and diagnostic methods to identify individuals at high medical and/or nutritional risk and provide interventions in the form of one-on-one counseling or small group counseling and education as part of a clinic or healthcare facility.

Community. Group of persons whose members share a common bond such as living in the same geographic area or sharing the same culture or language.

Community Assessment. Formal process of collecting and evaluating relevant information about the ecology of a particular community and applying the data to determine met and unmet needs of the community.

Community Health Services. Health services provided for a specific group of people who have a common bond such as language, geographic area, socioeconomic needs, or similar health problems.

Healthcare Team. A group of health professionals who work together with the common objective of providing comprehensive and coordinated healthcare services to individuals and their families.

Nutrition Assessment. Evaluation of the nutritional status of individuals or groups based on anthropometric, biochemical, clinical, and dietary information.

Population-Based Focus. Epidemiologic methods to describe health and nutrition needs in the community that serve as the basis for designing interventions to reach the general population or large segments of the population at particular risk.

Program Planning. The process by which administrators assess needs and develop a plan to meet these needs.

REFERENCES

1. ADA. "Position of the American Dietetic Association: The Roles of Registered Dietitians and Dietetic Technicians, Registered, in Health Promotion and Disease Prevention." *J Am Diet Assoc* 106(2006): 1875–1884.
2. Public Health Nutrition Practice Group of the American Dietetic Association. "Guidelines for Community Nutrition Supervised Practice Experience." The American Dietetic Association: Chicago; 2003.
3. Kaufman, M. *Nutrition in Public Health: A Handbook for Developing Programs and Services.* Aspen Publishers: Rockville, MD; 1990.
4. Institute of Medicine. "The Future of Public Health." Washington, D.C.: National Academy Press; 1989, p. 15.
5. Association of Graduate Programs in Public Health Nutrition, Inc. *Strategies for Success: Curriculum Guide for Graduate Programs in Public Health Nutrition.* Washington, D.C.: Association of the Faculties of Graduate Programs in Public Health Nutrition; 1990.
6. See Note 3.
7. Ibid.
8. American Dietetic Association. Compensation and Benefits Survey 2009. www.eatright.org. Accessed October 20, 2009.
9. See Note 2.
10. Dodds, J.M. and M. Kaufman. *Personnel in Public Health Nutrition for the 1990s: A Comprehensive Guide.* Washington, D.C.: The Public Health Foundation; 1991, p. 202.

CHAPTER 9

The Consultant in Health Care, Business, and Private Practice

"Many dietitians are doing what has not been done before. They embody the entrepreneurial spirit, their ingenuity, creative verve, and aggressiveness are leading them and the dietetics profession into new fields of experience."[1]

OUTLINE

- Introduction
- Becoming a Consultant
  - Contracts and Fees
- The Consultant in Health Care and Extended Care
  - Regulations
  - Areas of Practice
  - Roles and Responsibilities
  - Standards for Quality Assurance
- The Consultant in Business Practice
  - Areas of Practice
- The Dietitian in Private Practice
  - Starting a Practice
  - Areas of Practice
  - Practice Roles
- Ethical and Legal Bases of Practice
- Summary

INTRODUCTION

In the 2009 Compensation and Benefits Survey, it was reported that 8 percent of RDs and about 3 percent of DTRs indicated their primary practice area was in consultation and business.[2] Many dietitians have found the schedule flexibility and compensation of self-employment attractive alternatives to more traditional positions. An entrepreneurial drive is often the impetus for a professional to become a consultant or to establish his or her own practice, although many do so because family or other obligations demand a better lifestyle fit.

Healthcare institutions have moved an increasing number of services from inpatient care into outpatient clinics, other community agencies, or home care. Governmental regulations led to the need for nutrition consultants in extended care facilities. Together, both these trends have led to the need for a greater number of consultants rather than full-time employees.

Three types of consultant practice are discussed in this chapter: consultants in health care and extended care, consultants in business practice, and dietitians in private practice.

BECOMING A CONSULTANT

Starting a practice as a consultant requires forethought and planning. Two excellent publications available to guide the dietitian in planning are Helm's *The Competitive Edge* and *The Entrepreneurial Nutritionist*.[3,4] The first step is a self-assessment. Personal characteristics are important because an entrepreneur needs to be self-directed, energetic, and action-oriented. Previous working experience in dietetics is recommended for the person considering becoming a consultant because a great deal of independent activity and judgment is needed, and success is dependent on having had opportunity to develop these characteristics. A list of questions that can be used to determine readiness to enter practice alone is shown in Table 9-1.

Once the decision has been made to start a consulting practice, several actions need to be taken. If an office is established, appropriate office equipment must be obtained and decisions made about secretarial and/or office manager assistance. Networking with other successful dietitians through one or more practice groups is an excellent way of gaining valuable start-up information. Mentors may be found and networks estab-

Table 9-1. Questionnaire to Determine Readiness for Private Practice

Are you a self-starter?

3—I do things on my own—nobody has to tell me what to do or when to get started.

2—If someone gets me started, I keep going by myself.

1—Easy does it! Keep prodding me and I will move along fine.

Are you a risk taker?

3—I'll take a chance, even if I am unsure of success.

2—I'll jump in, if I am fairly sure of succeeding.

1—Uncertainty is not for me—I'll wait until success is guaranteed.

Do you have a positive, friendly interest in others?

3—I enjoy new people and can get along with just about anybody.

2—I am most comfortable with existing friends and don't need anyone else.

1—Meeting new people is not my forte. I prefer being alone.

Are you a leader?

3—I can get most people to go along when I start something.

2—I can give the orders if someone else tells 'me what we should do.

1—I let someone else get things moving, then I go along if I feel like it.

Can you handle responsibility?

3—I like to take charge of things and see them through.

2—I'll take over if I have to, but I'd rather let someone else be responsible.

1—I would rather not have the final responsibility.

Are you a good organizer?

3—I like to make plans and check them off; I like to get things going.

2—I do all right until things get too confused. Then I quit.

1—Things get done as they come. I don't like too much structure.

Are you prepared to put in as many hours as necessary to get the job done?

3—I can keep going long and hard for something I want.

2—I'll work hard for a while, until I've had enough.

1—It will either happen or it won't, so I don't work myself to death.

Do you make up your mind quickly?

3—I can make up my mind in a hurry when I need to and it usually turns out okay.

2—I need time to decide, otherwise I may regret the decision.

1—I can't decide without considering all the details and discussing them with others.

Can people rely on you?

3—I say what I mean and I deliver—it's simpler that way.

2—I try to be on the level, but can't always deliver as needed.

1—People never really pay attention, so I just say whatever is easiest.

(continues)

Table 9-1. Questionnaire to Determine Readiness for Private Practice *(continued)*

Can you withstand reversals without quitting?

3—Once I've made up my mind, nothing stops me.

2—I usually finish what I start if it goes well.

1—If it doesn't go well, I see no reason to keep hammering away.

Total your score. If your score is 24–30, you probably have what it takes to be in private practice. If your score is 17–23, running a business of your own would likely be an uphill battle. A total score below 16 suggests that you may not be ready to be independent in business.

Source: Cross, A.T. "Practical and Legal Considerations of Private Nutrition Practice." *J Am Diet Assoc* 95(1995): 21–29.

lished from these contacts. Consider professional liability insurance early in the planning stage. This insurance is available through the American Dietetic Association.

The consultant often locates "accounts" or positions through networking. Initiating contacts with facilities followed by interviews with the administrator and meeting other key personnel should occur. Negotiations should include a clear understanding of the amount of time the consultant will be needed. Although regulations in a healthcare facility may require a dietetic consultant only a minimum number of hours per month, there may be compelling reasons for more time to be spent in the facility. For instance, in institutions with a large number of residents or institutions in which a number of residents require skilled care, additional consultation time will be needed.

Contracts and Fees

Major considerations for the dietitian in consultation and private practice are setting prices and fees and obtaining reimbursement for services. A contract should specify the services to be provided, the amount of time allotted for the services, and fees to be assessed. Establishing and negotiating the ground rules are important in the initial stages of the process.[5]

Consultants can gain information about reimbursement rates by researching pay levels in the area and region for different types of consulting work and for basic salary levels. Networking with others in a practice group is a very good way of obtaining information regarding typical fees. Dietitians who receive reimbursement from insurers or hospitals for medical nutrition therapy (MNT) will be guided by MNT codes in establishing payment for treatments authorized by Medicare.[6]

Expenses such as liability insurance, mileage and travel expenses, and any educational components needed should be added in to arrive at a fee. A helpful discussion on the process of setting fees is presented in *The Entrepreneurial Nutritionist.*[7]

THE CONSULTANT IN HEALTH CARE AND EXTENDED CARE

The role of the consultant in healthcare facilities and extended care became important in the 1960s with the enactment of the Medicare regulations by the Health Care Financing Administration (now Centers for Medicare and Medicaid Services, or CMS). The Omnibus Reconciliation Act of 1987[8] published regulations for nutritional care in long-term facilities that received federal Medicare funds. These facilities (primarily nursing homes) were required to hire a qualified dietitian; as a result, the demand for consultant dietitians rapidly increased. From a limited employment area with a short history, few guidelines, and dietitians "on their own" insofar as job requirements and benefits were concerned, consultation in healthcare facilities became an arena in which many dietitians soon found positions. These opportunities helped many dietitians who had been out of the workforce for periods of time return to practice. Some of these dietitians needed to be updated in practice knowledge and skills and turned to continuing education opportunities to gain the necessary information to practice. Today, many dietitians work as consultants in nursing homes and small hospitals funded by federal and state agencies.

The amount of time a dietitian is needed is not specified in federal regulations. Instead, the regulations state that the consultant's visits should be of "sufficient frequency to meet the food and nutrition needs of the facility."[9] State licensing requirements, however, frequently specify a minimum of 8 hours per month. A dietitian contracts with a facility for the amount of time needed, at or above the minimum, to meet the facility's needs.

Many consultants are employed on a part-time basis in one or more facilities, although the individual's commitment could be full-time, depending on the number of facilities in which the consultant works and the amount of time he or she chooses to work. Some dietitians are employed full-time for a multifacility chain or in one large facility.

Regulations

A consultant must be familiar with state and federal regulations that apply to long-term or extended care facilities. The health department in each state can provide copies of both regulations. Federal regulations are precise concerning both the physical plant and the operation and staffing of the facility. Each facility has its own procedures and set of regulations governing operation. The consultant needs to be thoroughly familiar with these as well as the policies and goals of the facility.

All healthcare providers need to be familiar with the American Health Insurance Portability and Accountability Act (HIPAA) of 1996 as this set of rules concerning rights of patients and clients must be addressed, and clients notified of the consultant's privacy procedures.[10]

Areas of Practice

Long-term facilities include nursing homes, skilled nursing facilities, subacute care centers, adult daycare, residential care facilities, and alcohol and drug rehabilitation facilities. Long-term care facilities may be owned privately, by the city or county, by religious organizations, or by corporations. They may be for-profit or not-for-profit and may range in size from 50 to 200 beds or more.

Consultants also may be hired to visit developmentally disabled clients in their homes. In addition, some state health departments contract with consultants to provide services for Women, Infants, and Children (WIC) program participants. Other consultants work in home health care, congregate feeding sites, senior citizen centers, correctional facilities, group homes for the developmentally disabled, hospice programs, and small rural hospitals. Adult daycare, group homes, and retirement communities are other facilities offering opportunity for the consultant dietitian in health care.

Roles and Responsibilities

A consultant primarily functions in an advisory capacity within a facility; however, he or she has ethical and professional responsibilities for the nutritional care of the residents. By developing rapport and using organizational skills, the consultant is able to accomplish the needed tasks. Because he or she is usually not in the facility full-time, the day-to-day supervision of the facility may be provided by a dietetic manager or technician.

When a consultant begins employment in a facility, one of the first activities should be a needs assessment in food service and nutrition services for the residents. This assessment will guide further planning and action. Documentation of observations and plans for future visits is very important, beginning with the first visit. The typical activities a consultant performs during a visit to the facility may include the following:[11]

- Confer with the dietary manager and the administrator about day-to-day operations and any problems that need to be addressed during the visit.
- Perform nutrition assessments of new residents and conduct a follow-up for all others.
- Check at-risk residents and make recommendations for further nutritional care as indicated. This includes noting unexplained changes in weight or the development of pressure ulcers, checking those on tube feedings, and noting signs of dehydration or otherwise poor nutritional status.[12,13]
- Observe the meal service and eat a meal to evaluate food quality.
- Make nutrition rounds at meal time to observe the residents' acceptance of the food and their food intake.
- Conduct educational in-service sessions for employees and exchange information regarding departmental activities.
- Document all activities with any recommendations for follow-up.

The consultant may be responsible for developing policy and procedure manuals for the quality improvement program, for safety and sanitation procedures, and for budget management. The reference diet manual should be reviewed and signed by the chief of the medical staff at least annually and should be updated regularly. Consultants may also teach dietetic technician students, conduct classes for dietary managers, and serve as preceptors for students in supervised experiences in long-term care.

Standards for Quality Assurance

The Consultant Dietitians in Health Care Facilities dietetic practice group (now the Dietitians in Health Care Communities) developed standards of practice in 2001 as a guide for quality assurance.[14] The standards specify six areas of activity, with examples of outcomes. They include provision of services, application of research, communication and application of knowledge, utilization and management of resources, and continued competence and professional accountability.

Through written documentation, consultant dietitians can verify actual performance and implement action to meet the expected outcomes. The standards also help dietitians develop a workable plan to meet the responsibilities for which they have contracted and to evaluate their own knowledge, clinical experience, and management expertise.

THE CONSULTANT IN BUSINESS PRACTICE

An increasingly popular area of practice for the dietitian with an entrepreneurial drive is in business and nontraditional career areas. Potential practice areas identified by the Nutrition Entrepreneur practice group of the ADA include services for individuals, corporations, the media, restaurants, food companies, Internet and business technology, sports and health facilities, and coaching. Other areas are in pharmaceutical sales, medical and institutional equipment sales, catering, chefs' schools, and specialized clinics.

Dietitians who work as consultants in businesses of all kinds like to take on new challenges and are often described as risk-takers in new areas of practice. They are energetic and versatile individuals with background experience preparing them for innovative roles—roles they may even be required to create. Although many of the responsibilities of a consultant may be similar to those for a full-time dietitian, one of the main differences is often the duration of the assignment. In an established business, the consultant may be given a short-term contract with an identified scope. The scope of services is usually an assignment to set up or improve the business practices of the client. It also may be a specific project with a defined beginning and end time period. Examples of activities the consultant may perform include evaluating staffing patterns, establishing an inventory and cost control system, planning a new production or service system, recommending equipment purchase, or establishing a computerized control system.

Areas of Practice

Business consulting firms at times employ entry-level dietitians for consulting, but usually in a defined scope of responsibility. More often, the dietitian is experienced in some area (e.g., as a clinical dietitian in a healthcare facility or manager of a food service system). The dietitian also may have worked as an assistant to another dietitian for a food processor, equipment manufacturer, publisher, marketing company, or software specialist. When hired, he or she may first be assigned to a team leader to work on a specific part of a major project. With experience, there may be opportunities to expand into other nontraditional roles such as facility management, accounting, design, sales, or marketing. The range of expanded responsibility is dependent on the scope of the services performed by the company and those that the dietitian can develop for the company.

The following guidelines are proposed for those who may be thinking of moving into management with the goal of consultation as his or her own business.

- Consider one's personal qualifications to act independently.
- Seek advice from a veteran manager or other mentors.
- React deliberately rather than spontaneously.
- Weigh solutions against the mission of the organization.
- Practice active listening with everyone involved.
- Keep up-to-date with the professional literature and continuing education opportunities, and consider further education if advancement and pay would benefit.

THE DIETITIAN IN PRIVATE PRACTICE

Many dietitians today become entrepreneurs and enter private practice for a variety of reasons. Some seek new and innovative opportunities out of choice; others do so due to circumstances that make private practice a viable option. Examples of the latter might be the loss of a job or the need to work varying hours because of family responsibilities. Opportunities for women in the business world are unquestionably increasing. The healthcare industry continues to downsize from large centralized centers to outpatient and community centers with fewer staff. Many dietitians seek greater independence and new challenges and, along with a business climate that encourages entrepreneurs, find satisfying careers in private practice.[15]

Not all entrepreneurs start a business as described. Some work at home and may combine home and family responsibilities with part-time, contract-type work, including consulting, writing, computer searches, home visits, and so forth. Others may open an office, hire assistants, and establish a full-time practice or business.

Starting a Practice

Cross[16] provides a helpful checklist for getting started in private practice. The first step, she points out, is to maintain an updated file of one's professional credentials and achievements. Regarding references, both giving and receiving employment references may present important issues to be considered.[17] Obtaining state licensure or certification and keeping professional credentials up-to-date helps establish qualifications. Secondly, joining the state association, dietetic practice groups, and specialty groups, if applicable, will provide opportunities for networking. Becoming involved in local business groups or taking business classes helps one learn the business climate.

Creating a vision and finding one's focus, then creating the roadmap, or business plan, is the next step.[18] The business plan includes an executive summary, description of the company along with the mission and vision statements, product or service, a description of the target market, the competition, and financial projections. A professional support system consisting of an accountant, a banker, a marketing specialist, an information technology specialist, and perhaps a lawyer, will all provide valuable assistance. As Norton[19] points out, depending on the person's business organization, mentors, partners, and a Board of Directors also may be needed as the business proceeds. Banks and investment companies often provide advice also and assist entrepreneurs in starting a business.

Establishing the business basics by estimating expenses, obtaining necessary insurance, setting up and staffing an office, and writing basic business policies and procedures are the next steps. After this, a marketing and a quality-assurance program will help launch and maintain the business.[20] The benefits that can be realized from careful planning include seeing clients succeed and realizing a business profit.

The dietitian who enters private practice needs to possess several qualities, such as confidence, determination, perseverance, and the motivation to remain current on trends and changes in the profession. Remaining up-to-date comes in great part through taking advantage of continuing education opportunities. The Nutrition Entrepreneurs Group advises that anyone going into private practice, whether to write a book, start a business, become a speaker or coach, or use the Internet to market or provide

products and services, will find help through a mentor and offers participation in a mentorship program.

Areas of Practice

The consultant in private practice will usually be located outside an organization, but also may be an "intrapreneur," or one within an organization, who develops new ideas or services that are used profitably in some
way. The potential work settings are as diverse as the practitioner's interests
and expertise, as well as the market demands. This variety is illustrated in
Table 9-2.

The professional services provided are influenced by the needs of the
consumer, the demands and changing environments of health care,
changes in regulatory agencies, increased autonomy, and advances in science and technology.[21] As new ideas are disseminated and needs identified, more roles are defined for the private practitioner. Dietitians may
form alliances and networks to provide services. By teaming with other
professionals, the ability to market services and products and share business expense is enhanced. The opportunities presented through a wider
range of contacts also may be increased. Examples of such associations are

Table 9-2. Settings for Consulting in Private Practice

Private office	Media and communications
Private home	Grocery stores
Physician or other allied health professional offices	Restaurant and culinary industry
	Corporate settings of worksites
Home health care	Business and industry
Health/fitness centers and spas	Food companies
Community-based programs	Hotels and resorts
Schools	Research centers
Hospitals	Medical education consulting firms
Day homes	Private specialty clinics (sports medi-
Senior citizen centers	cine, eating disorders, diabetes,
Nursing homes	renal, oncology, HIV/AIDS)
Contracts with government agencies	Rehabilitation centers

Source: Alexander-Israel, D. and C. Roman-Shriver. In *Dietetics: Practice and Future Trends.*
E.A. Winterfeldt, M.L. Bogle, and L.L. Ebro. Aspen Publishers: Gaithersburg, MD; 1998,
p. 208.

preferred provider organizations to managed care companies, dietitian networks, and dietitian-independent practice associations.[22] Dietetic practice groups in the ADA provide a means for networking to occur among professionals.

Practice Roles

Consultants in private practice may teach clients and consumers in areas ranging from wellness and prevention to medical nutrition therapy, business and industry, education and training, food service and culinary trades, and writing and media presentation. A list of activities is shown in Table 9-3 as examples of the types of services that consultants may perform.

Table 9-3. Roles of Consultants in Private Practice

Assessment of nutritional status

Menu evaluation and planning

Recipe evaluation and modification

One-on-one counseling

Family counseling

Group counseling

Monitoring of nutritional intervention

Dietary analysis and evaluation of products

Consultant to agencies, institutions, and programs with nutrition components, such as extended care, school food service, hospitals, government agencies, or clinics

Consultant to professionals (health care, food service, culinary industry)

Consultant to corporations (fitness centers, wellness/health promotion programs, benefits departments)

Writing for the lay public (books, newsletters, magazines, newspaper articles)

Professional publications

Group training, presentations, workshops

Developing nutritious/healthier menu items for restaurants

Restaurant and culinary staff training

Assistance in marketing nutrition in restaurants

Computer/software programming (quality management, nutrition education, food service, clinical nutrition)

Developing and marketing nutrition education programs (private and public)

Supermarket tours and grocery information guides

Nutrition labeling information

(continues)

Table 9-3. Roles of Consultants in Private Practice *(continued)*

Rehabilitation and sports injury consultation
Nutrition care planning
Monitoring compliance with local, state, federal regulations (long-term care facilities, drug and alcohol centers, prisons)
Developing, administering, and evaluating nutrition standards
Multidisciplinary preventive and therapeutic services
Health coaching

Source: Alexander-Israel, D. and C. Roman-Shriver In *Dietetics: Practice and Future Trends.* E.A. Winterfeldt, M.L. Bogle, and L.L. Ebro. Aspen Publishers: Gaithersburg, MD; 1998, p. 209.

Practice roles often can be expanded with more training in business, marketing, and communications and with the development of new skills that cross the boundaries into other health professionals.[23] For example, dietitians can become proficient at taking blood pressure and body composition measurements in the home care setting; can secure American College of Sports Medicine Exercise Test Technology certification for performing electrocardiogram-monitored stress tests in sports medicine clinics, Clinical Laboratory Improvement Certification for blood analysis; or can use phlebotomy skills in wellness programs.

Continually emerging roles demand expansion of the dietitian's scope of practice and skills and capitalizing on the talents that are unique to dietitians. Among these are the ability to apply food and nutrition knowledge, use nutrition assessment tools, apply lifestyle-change education to prevent or manage disease, and to collect data on outcomes of nutrition intervention on quality of life and overall care costs.

ETHICAL AND LEGAL BASES OF PRACTICE

Important guides for the dietitian are the professional code of conduct and any applicable rule or statute of practice from the state and local authorities under whose jurisdiction the dietitian practices. These documents will clarify disciplinary action that can be taken by the professional or regulatory agencies on violations of the code, covering such activities as advertising and practicing medicine versus nutrition. Feeney[24] offers very practical tips for the dietitian applying the code of ethics to ethical practice when questions or conflicts arise. Along the same lines, the advice of an attorney is indispensable relative to business law and limits on the private practice of nutrition and the laws of the state in which the practice is established.

SUMMARY

Traditional institutional roles for dietitians, especially in clinical dietetics, are still predominant practice settings; however, many dietitians are using their clinical background to become entrepreneurs in their own practice. The dietitian who possesses the needed personal attributes and the initiative and creativity needed for entrepreneurial success may find a rewarding new career in consultation in healthcare facilities, business, or private practice.

DEFINITIONS

Client. The recipient of services or products.

Consultant. A skilled or knowledgeable person qualified to give expert professional advice.

Continuous Quality Improvement. The continued study and improvement of the process and outcomes of healthcare services to meet the needs of those served. Specific structured problem-solving methods are used that rely on data and group process tools.

Intrapraneur. A person within an organization who develops new ideas or services.

Long-Term Care. Assistance provided over time to people with chronic health conditions and/or physical disabilities and those who are unable to care for themselves.

Managed Care. A system of health care administered by an entity outside a hospital or healthcare institution in which access, cost, and quality of care are controlled by direct intervention before or during service for purposes of creating efficiencies and/or reducing costs.

Nutrition Assessment. Evaluation of an individual's nutritional status based on anthropometric, biochemical, clinical, and dietary information.

Nutrition Screening. The use of diagnostic methodology to determine nutritional risk and the necessity of an in-depth nutrition assessment.

Private Practice. Self-employment in which a person manages his or her own working career.

Subacute Care. Services provided in a treatment unit, usually after acute hospital care and before home care or a long-term care facility.

REFERENCES

1. Helm, K.K. *The Entrepreneurial Nutritionist.* 2nd ed. K.K. Helm Publications: Lake Dallas, TX; 1991, p. 1
2. American Dietetic Association. Compensation and Benefits Survey of the Dietetic Profession 2009. www.eatright.org. Accessed October 15, 2009.
3. Helm, K.K. *The Competitive Edge: Advanced Marketing for Dietetic Professionals.* The American Dietetic Association: Chicago; 1995.
4. See Note 1.
5. McCafree, J. "Contract Basics: What a Dietitian Should Know." *J Am Diet Assoc* 103, no. 4(2003): 429–440.
6. Bender, T. "2009 Medicare MNT Payment Information." *Ventures* (Publication of Nutrition Entrepreneurs Practice group) XXV, no. 4(2009): 10.
7. See Note 1.
8. Robinson, G. and C. Russell. "OBRA Regulations Revisited." *Diet Curric* 23(1996): 15–20.
9. "Skilled Nursing Facilities: Standards for Certification and Participation in Medicare and Medicaid Programs." *Federal Register* 39(1974):22–38.
10. "Health Insurance Portability and Accountability Act." 1996. www.hhs.gov (Accessed April 24, 2009).
11. Nichols, P. "The Consultant in Health Care Facilities/Extended Care." In *Dietetics: Practice and Future Trends.* E.A. Winterfeldt, M.L. Bogle, and L.L. Ebro. Aspen Publishers: Gaithersburg, MD; 1998, p. 222.
12. Chidester, J.C. and A.A. Spangler. "Fluid Intake in the Institutionalized Elderly." *J Am Diet Assoc* 97(1997): 23–27.
13. White J.V., R.J. Ham, D.A. Lipschitz, and J.Y. Dwyer. "Consensus of the Nutrition Screening Initiative: Risk Factors and Indicators of Poor Nutritional Status in Older Americans." *J Am Diet Assoc* 91(1991): 783–787.
14. Vogelsang, J.L. and L.L. Roth-Yousey. "Standards of Professional Practice: Measuring the Beliefs and Realities of Consultant Dietitians in Health Care Facilities." *J Am Diet Assoc* 101, no. 49(2001): 473–480.
15. Rejent-Scholtz, A. "The Growth of Entrepreneurship." In *The Competitive Edge: Advanced Marketing for Dietetic Professionals.* The American Dietetic Association: Chicago; 1995, pp. 8–10.

16. Cross, M. "Getting Started in Private Practice: A Checklist to Your Entrepreneurial Path." *J Am Diet Assoc* 108, no. 1(2008): 21–24.

17. Zackin, F.M. "Employment References—Giving and Receiving." *J Am Diet Assoc* 108, no. 6(2008): 1053–1055.

18. Peregrin, T. "Business Plan 2.0: Putting Technology to Work." *J Am Diet Assoc* 108, no. 2(2008): 212–214.

19. Norton, L.C. "The Consultant in Business Practice." In *Dietetics: Practice and Future Trends.* E.A. Winterfeldt, M.L. Bogle, and L.L. Ebro. Aspen Publishers: Gaithersburg, MD; 1998, p. 236.

20. Mathieu, J. "Marketing Yourself and Taking Risks." *J Am Diet Assoc* 109, no. 1(2009): 28–29.

21. ADA. "The Role of Dietetics Professionals on Health Promotion and Disease Prevention." *J Am Diet Assoc* 102(2002): 1680–1687.

22. Israel, D. and S. Moores. *Beyond Nutrition Counseling: Achieving Positive Outcomes Through Nutrition Therapy.* Nutrition Entrepreneurs Dietetic Practice Group: Chicago; 1996, p. 14.

23. See Note 19.

24. Feeney, M.J. "When Ethics Collide: An Independent Dietetic Consultant's Perspective on Balancing Professional Ethics with the Wishes of Your Client. *J Am Diet Assoc* 108, no. 1(2008): 29–31.

CHAPTER 10

Career Choices in Business, Education, and Health and Wellness

"The ancient Greeks attained a high level of civilization based on good nutrition, regular physical activity, and intellectual development."[1]

OUTLINE

- Introduction
- The Dietitian in Business and Communications
  - Career Opportunities
  - Mentors and Networks
  - Strategic Skill Building
- The Dietitian in Health and Wellness Programs
  - Sports Nutrition
  - Cardiovascular Nutrition
  - Wellness and Health Promotion
  - Disordered Eating
- The Dietitian in Education and Research
  - The Dietitian in Education
  - The Dietitian in Research
  - Career Preparation
  - Education and Research Practice Groups
- Summary

INTRODUCTION

Hospitals and extended care facilities are the work settings for the largest percentage of dietitians and dietetic technicians; however, there are many career choices available in other settings to both the entry-level and the experienced professional. Consultation and private practice were discussed in Chapter 9. In this chapter, three areas of dietetics practice opportunity are presented: business and communications, education and research, and health and wellness programs.

THE DIETITIAN IN BUSINESS AND COMMUNICATIONS

Following a career path in business and communications has long been considered a nontraditional choice for dietitians. The ADA membership survey in 2009[2] shows that about 30 percent of dietitians work in the for-profit sector, including those in contract food management, managed care organizations, and other for-profit organizations. This for-profit category also represents a wide range of positions, including private practice and working with corporations, trade associations, food and pharmaceutical companies, and hotels and restaurants.

Expanded opportunities in business and communications are expected to continue and grow as employers add dietitians to their organization. Major reasons appear to be to increase the company's credibility, to promote customer health and nutrition, and to increase the understanding of customer needs. Given the current trends reported by the Food Marketing Institute,[3] in *Trends—Consumer Attitudes and the Supermarket,* most consumers believe their diets could be more healthful and they are taking more responsibility for ensuring that what they eat is nutritious. Although taste remains the number one criterion when choosing food (89% studied considered it very important), nutrition and product safety (79% each) were rated very important in food selection. Food producers, food retailers, and food service establishments take note of these trends and respond to meet what the consuming public wants.

Career Opportunities

There are many paths to a career in business and communications for the interested and qualified dietitian (Table 10-1). The importance of early exposure to the business world is increasingly recognized, as pointed out in recommendations that dietetics students experience a rotation in a business environment as part of their undergraduate, dietetic internship, or graduate study.[4] Students and supervisors can discover opportunities by contacting exhibitors at professional meetings, local businesses, or by contacting other professionals in business and communications. A business rotation may also offer opportunity for exposure to marketing and public relations activities that are essential in business.

The Dietitians in Business and Communications practice group identify their members as presidents, vice presidents, food service directors,

Table 10-1. Career Opportunities in Business and Communications

Food Industry
  Food and beverage manufacturing and distributing
  Market research companies
  Trade associations
  Hotels and restaurants
  Contract food service companies
  Commodity groups such as the pork, beef, and egg producers
  National associations
    National Dairy Association
    National Livestock and Meat Board
    Food Marketing Institute
    Grocery Manufacturers
Communications
  Freelance writing
  Writing for publications or newsletters
  Public relations and advertising
  Media spokesperson
  Computer training
  Internet education and services
Health Industry Groups
  Worksite wellness programs
  Health clubs and spas
  Pharmaceutical companies
  Nutritional product and dietary supplement companies
  Heart, cancer, and diabetes associations

food stylists, researchers, consultants, sales manager, marketing managers, restauranteurs, test kitchen managers, and software specialists.

How does an individual get a start in business? Several steps are important:[5]

- Make a list of your talents and interests.
- Make a list of all the possible areas into which you could work, including, but not limited to, writing, speaking, publishing, research, marketing, teaching, sales, media, cooking demonstrations, counseling, coaching, managing, catering, and product development.
- Make a list of the populations with whom you enjoy working.
- Read newsletters—the ADA journal, dietetic practice group newsletters, and other publications—and make a list of dietitians doing things you would enjoy doing.
- Contact those working in areas of interest.
- Network, network, network!

Dietitians in business and communications cite several positive things they like about their jobs: challenging work, learning opportunities, opportunity for creativity, fast pace, visibility, and remuneration. At the same time, some indicate there can be stress, long hours, a fast pace, bureaucracy, and a lot of information to absorb. The dietitian who is flexible and experienced in the business world is most likely to succeed.

Mentors and Networks

Dietitians traveling a nontraditional path agree that having a mentor, networking, developing a strategic skill set, and keeping current with research and consumer trends are factors necessary to build a successful career. A mentor may be a coworker, an instructor, or another professional. A mentor in the same organization can provide insight into policies, procedures, and the unspoken policies of a company.

Networking both inside and outside the boundaries of dietetics is a way of finding a mentor, gathering information, and connecting with others.[6] The networking offered through DPGs is invaluable to professionals looking for opportunities for change or advancement in nontraditional areas. Affiliating with other professional associations will provide more ideas and contacts.

Strategic Skill Building

The ability to communicate effectively, along with business savvy and public relations, or "people" skills, is strategic to a successful career. Industry studies routinely point out that communicating well means the difference between success and failure. The ability to build on earlier education and experiences leads to professional growth and enhanced job performance. For example, if a job requires evaluating research and working with research and development, a good grounding in science is important. Clinical education and experience help a dietitian understand the health and nutritional implications when producing and marketing a new food or supplement or educational materials.

Advancing into positions with greater responsibility and managerial-skill requirements may necessitate continuing education, often in the business-related areas of study. The growth of online and distance education helps make this possible even for the professional working full-time or in locations away from the educational setting. Dietitians in business frequently continue their education by acquiring an MBA or an advanced degree in management or finance.

Dietitians in business often establish a Web site in order to improve their business image, complement business advertising, attract new clients or customers outside the local area, or to start a new business venture.[7] They may also find this a useful way to learn more about specific businesses and to build networks.

THE DIETITIAN IN HEALTH AND WELLNESS PROGRAMS

Wellness, health promotion, corporate fitness, and sports nutrition programs are all career areas that have developed in recent years. Although both sports and dietetics as professions or areas of interest have existed for centuries, the combination of the two as a career specialty is relatively recent. The growth of wellness and fitness programs has been rapid as the relationship between nutritional status and maintenance of health and prevention of disease becomes more evident.[8]

Diet is a known risk factor for the development of the three chronic diseases that are the leading cause of death in adults in the United States: cancer, cardiovascular disease, and stroke.[9] Additional health problems of adults are also closely associated with diet and eating behaviors: obesity, diabetes, high blood pressure, and osteoporosis. The numbers of deaths and medical costs can be significantly altered by changes in diet and lifestyle when it is considered that billions of dollars are spent each year on schemes and gimmicks to reduce body weight and prevent cancer, not to mention the money spent treating adults with these diseases and their complications.

Reports from the National Health and Nutrition Examination Survey III (NHANES III) indicate an alarming increase in the prevalence and severity of obesity in young children, older children, and adolescents, as well as adults.[10] These statistics and research point to the need for programs in health promotion, wellness, fitness, and the prevention and treatment of obesity, which greatly expands career options for dietitians.

Some dietitians have developed their own programs through practice and research and now market or license the programs to other dietitians and health professionals, both nationally and internationally. Others continue to work in hospitals, ambulatory care centers, clinics, rehabilitation centers, and athletic clubs or gyms. Those in private practice provide counseling and medical nutrition therapies aimed at preventing and treating obesity.

Even with, or perhaps because of, the increasing prevalence of obesity, many dietary fads, drugs, and questionable dieting programs have escalated and consume enormous amounts of money each year. This phenomenon emphasizes the need and opportunities that exist for dietitians and other health professionals in this area.

Sports Nutrition

Interest in sports and cardiovascular nutrition among members of the ADA led to the formation in 1981 of the Sports and Cardiovascular Nutritionists (SCAN) DPG of nutrition professionals within the ADA. In 1993, SCAN changed its name to "Sports, Cardiovascular and Wellness Nutritionists" to reflect the importance of wellness and health promotion as a growing areas of dietetic practice. In 1994, SCAN welcomed dietetic professionals with an interest in disordered eating into its fold, recognizing the frequent presence of eating disorders among athletes and the critical role that the identification and treatment of disordered eating has in maintaining health and wellness.

The ADA, the Canadian Association, and the American College of Sports Nutrition issued a position paper in 2000 concerning nutrition and athletic performance.[11] The importance of optimal nutrition and the roles and responsibilities of healthcare professionals were discussed in the paper. The educational needs of those aspiring to be sports nutritionists were detailed in an article by Clark.[12] Nutrition knowledge, exercise science knowledge, business skills, and a foundation of strong clinical experience are all important, especially because many sports nutritionists are entrepreneurs. A list of the clinical concerns commonly presented to a sports nutritionist is shown in Table 10-2.

Dietetic professionals with a specialty in sports nutrition can be found in a wide variety of settings, from sports medicine clinics to professional football teams, from high school athletics to the Olympics, and from universities to fitness centers. Many incorporate sports nutrition into their more general practice of nutrition counseling or private practice. Today, several professional sports teams include dietitians as paid consultants whose expertise serves to enhance the players' performance. A few professional athletes have employed personal dietitians primarily to help them maintain appropriate body weight and ratio of fat to lean body mass.

Some dietitians serve as nutrition trainers for college athletes and teams that specialize in the sport or sports in which they have the greatest personal interest, such as swimming, wrestling, baseball, cycling, and others.

The duties and work settings of a sports nutritionist are many and varied and often require irregular work hours such as evenings and weekends.

Table 10-2. Clinical Concerns Commonly Presented to a Sports Nutritionist

Allergies	Gastric reflux
Alcohol addiction	Gout
Amenorrhea	Headaches
Anemia	Hypoglycemia
Anorexia	Hyperlipidemia
Arteriosclerosis	Hypertension
Binge eating	Menopause
Body image distortion	Obesity/overweight
Bulimia	Osteoporosis
Cancer (prevention, recovery from)	Pregnancy/perinatal nutrition
Chronic fatigue	Stress fractures
Constipation	Surgery (special nutritional needs pre- and postoperative)
Diabetes	
Diarrhea	

Source: Clark, N. "Identifying the Educational Needs of Aspiring Sports Nutritionists." *J Am Diet Assoc* 100, no. 12(2000): 1522–1524.

A dietitian may occasionally need to travel with a sports team, and this travel may not always be funded by the team.

Many dietetic professionals working in the area of sports nutrition also work as a clinical dietitian for acute-care facilities, as outpatient dietitians, or in private practice in nutrition consulting. In addition, some dietitians are employed to supervise the food production and training table in college athletic residence halls. Some professional athletes seek information on diet during off-season to maintain body weight and strength. As part of his or her daily routine, a sports nutritionist may counsel athletes one-on-one regarding their food intake and appropriate nutrients or their use of dietary supplemental aids.[13] A nutritionist may also conduct group classes on low-fat eating at a fitness center or work with a high school team to suggest healthful choices for eating when the team travels. Sports nutritionists also serve as part-time staff at health clubs, and are available to answer questions members may ask on nutrition or to conduct classes on eating for competition and good health.

An additional career for some dietitians with experience in sports nutrition and fitness has emerged in writing and developing nutrition education materials appropriate for athletes of all ages. Others may enjoy speaking and/or writing for the media and consultative arrangements with any number of organizations. Another career option that is growing emanates from the proliferation of gymnasiums and physical fitness centers for young children and adolescents. Although started for tumbling and gymnastic opportunities, it is becoming apparent that there is a need for expertise in nutrition in these settings, especially combined with the principles of child development. Parents and consumers are welcoming the dietitian's expertise related to obesity, weight maintenance, and disordered eating patterns in young children and adolescents. In some instances, entrepreneurial dietitians are developing centers and mobile units that go to elementary schools or other sites for demonstrations of appropriate physical activity and the benefits of good food choices and nutrition.

A knowledge of exercise physiology through coursework in exercise science is essential if the sports nutritionist combines nutrition and exercise in work with clients. Many dietetic professionals seek to enhance their education and expertise by entering graduate programs in exercise physiology, counseling psychology, or business administration. In addition, although few college or university programs in sports nutrition currently exist, many graduate students choose to conduct research for their thesis or dissertation on a topic directly related to sports nutrition. By acquiring a strong foundation in foods and normal and clinical nutrition with study in a related area, the dietetic student can better prepare him- or herself for practice in sports nutrition.

Cardiovascular Nutrition

With the abundance of research continuing in the area of diet and heart disease, as well as the fact that heart disease remains the number one cause of death for Americans, careers in cardiovascular nutrition offer abundant options. Most acute-care facilities whose services include open-heart surgery have cardiac rehabilitation programs in place. These typically include inpatient and outpatient components, both of which offer nutrition counseling and education as part of the program. Cardiac rehabilitation programs offer multidisciplinary teams who deal with all aspects of risk factor reduction, as well as education of the patient and family. Team members may include a medical director, cardiac rehabilitation nurse clinicians, exercise specialist, physical therapist, social worker, occupational therapist, and a dietitian. Education of the patient and family is often conducted in a variety of ways, from individual instruction to group classes. The dietitians may also design and conduct classes on low-fat cooking and other food preparation techniques.

Dietitians who specialize in cardiovascular nutrition may be employed by lipid research clinics. These professionals are responsible for teaching clinic patients how to change their eating habits to lower total fat and saturated fat or to comply with a research feeding protocol. In this setting at a university, they may conduct research on the latest cardiology protocols. Opportunities also exist with pharmaceutical companies as sales representatives or in the public relations departments of large food companies that market products to patients with cardiovascular disease and their families.

Wellness and Health Promotion

The opportunities for dietitians in wellness and health promotion are numerous and diverse. Dietitians who specialize in wellness may have a private practice or consulting business and negotiate contracts with industry, communities, or health clubs. Others are employed by medical centers or corporations to manage their on-site wellness and health promotion programs, which may include conducting classes for employees, developing incentives to foster a greater interest in exercise and nutrition, and increasing productivity by helping to reduce employee illness. Because nutrition is part of wellness, dietitians specializing in wellness and health promotion also may be involved in programs on smoking cessation, meditation and yoga, stress management, exercise, back safety, and employee relations.

Corporations and large institutions initially began providing worksite wellness programs for their employees because research and reports showed that these programs improved employee health, increased productivity, and decreased absenteeism and lost work days due to illness. As these programs developed and increased in numbers across the country in businesses of all sizes, data began to accumulate on the economic benefits of worksite wellness programs. With healthcare costs soaring and major changes occurring in healthcare and insurance coverages, employers were eager to explore wellness and health promotion programs that would save the corporation money. The common method for defining economic benefits is through the benefit-cost ratio in which the cost is the actual dollar cost of providing the program, and benefits are expressed in dollars saved from reduced absenteeism, disability expenses, and medical costs.

The ability to work as a facilitator and to conduct classes in a group setting is an important characteristic of the successful wellness professional. Counseling skills are also necessary because dealing with high-risk persons may be a regular aspect of the job. In addition, the dietitians must be prepared to analyze and evaluate enormous amounts of information available to employees and clients through media routes. This counseling may take place in groups, individually, at health fairs, or over the telephone.

Wellness and fitness programs are also emerging for the aging and retired population as well as the younger employed groups. Research indicates that even though aging is inevitable, biologic aging can be delayed through appropriate nutrition and exercise.[14] As the number of senior citizens increases, this will provide another career opportunity for dietitians specializing in health promotion. Fitness programs including nutrition, exercise, and lifestyle changes are developing that improve the quality of life and encourage wellness in this age group.

Several national organizations provide excellent and accurate information for dietitians seeking up-to-date knowledge on wellness and health promotion programs and concepts. In addition, all have information on the Internet. The major organizations with this information are the following:

- The American Dietetic Association (www.eatright.org)
- International Food Information Council (ificinfo.health.org)
- National Institutes of Health (www.nih.gov)
- President's Council on Physical Fitness and Sports (www.os.dhhs.gov)
- Centers for Disease Control and Prevention (www.cdc.gov)
- American College of Sports Medicine (www.csm.org)
- American Alliance on Health, Physical Education, Recreation, and Dance (www.ashperd.org)
- Food and Nutrition Information Center (www.fnic.nal.usda.gov)

The Internet also offers the opportunity and challenge for the individual dietitian to develop Web sites and disseminate nutrition and fitness messages by this means.

Disordered Eating

Dietitians who specialize in disordered eating work in a variety of settings, including residential treatment centers, hospitals (both medical and psychiatric), outpatient clinics, managed care organizations, university health centers, and private practice. The specialty of disordered or problematic eating encompasses several areas in which nutritional, physical, and psychological issues are intertwined with eating behavior, such as obesity, chronic dieting, anorexia nervosa, bulimia nervosa, compulsive eating, and binge eating disorders.[15] Complications of these disorders are potentially life threatening. Many have their origin or manifestation in childhood or adolescence. Although most of these disorders affect adolescent females, there have been some reports of similar behavior in males. Effective treatment of disordered eating requires knowledge and skills in counseling, cognitive behavioral therapy, family systems theory, addiction, and psychopharmacology.[16]

Because of the biopsychosocial nature of disordered eating, the role of the dietitian on the treatment team is vital. The dietitian educates the client about food, physical activity, and body size and shape and guides him or her in developing a sound eating style and physical activity pattern. Clients may share their thoughts and feelings about food, weight, and physical activity with the dietitian. They may also share life situations and events that are stressful for them, such as job change, marital problems, school problems, relationships, and burnout. The dietitian helps clients identify how stress affects their eating style and how they feel about food, their body size and shape, and physical activity. Ongoing communication with the treatment team therapist, psychiatrist, and physician is essential so that the dietitian can discern which issues are nutrition-related and which are psychological or medical. It takes years of experience for the dietitian to most effectively complement his or her skills and expertise with other members of the team.

Dietitians working in programs to treat disordered eating benefit from regular supervision from a mental health professional who specializes in problematic eating. This relationship provides a forum for discussion of specific cases, as well as helping to clarify which issues are appropriately addressed in nutrition therapy versus psychotherapy. Furthermore, many dietitians seek continuing education in areas such as women's issues, cognitive behavioral therapy, family counseling, psychotherapeutic counseling skills, and psychopharmacology. The intention is to sharpen counseling skills and enhance the understanding of sociological and psychological aspects of disordered eating while consistently staying within the scope of practice of the dietetic professional.

THE DIETITIAN IN EDUCATION AND RESEARCH

Almost every dietitian is an educator at least some of the time. For example, the dietitian in food service conducts in-service programs for employees, and public health nutritionists give classes for home care nurses as well as clients. Clinical dietitians participate in medical nutrition education, and they may conduct group classes for patients and families of those with diabetes, coronary heart disease, and so on. Dietitians working with WIC's food programs may teach Head Start children and parents how to prevent or reduce the incidence of obesity and adult-onset diabetes. Consultant dietitians may give food demonstrations for chefs and others. In industry, dietitians are called on to teach sales representatives and consumers about specialty nutrition products and to develop product materials for their clientele and the public. Many dietitians are preceptors for dietetics students and, as such, teach in both formal and informal ways, primarily in practice settings. Dietitians in every area of practice present information for clients and the public during National Nutrition Month in March. Because of the many opportunities that exist for dietitians to teach about their areas of expertise, it is essential that they are knowledgeable about and use principles of good teaching practices as discussed fully in Chapter 12.

Many dietitians conduct research as a part of their work. This is especially true for dietitians who specialize in nutrition support, pediatrics, renal dietetics, oncology, AIDS, diabetes, or other clinical subspecialties. These dietitians, and those in all other areas of practice, use research in various ways, may critique research, and collect research data for professional reference as needed. All dietitians are encouraged to perform or collect data for outcome research studies to demonstrate the effectiveness of medical nutrition therapy and/or the quality and acceptance of the services performed. In the clinical setting, dietitians may collaborate with physicians who are conducting nutrition-related studies, and even though they may not call themselves "researchers," they are in fact participating in research.

The Dietitian in Education

Elementary and Secondary Schools

Most school-based nutrition education is incorporated into health and science classes in primary, middle, and high schools. A dietitian who teaches at these levels must meet state teacher training and certification requirements. Generally, those who teach grades K–12 have responsibilities that extend well beyond food, nutrition, and health.

Some state departments of education have nutrition education and training sections that often employ Registered Dietitians who have advanced degrees in education. Such positions include creating curricula to integrate nutrition with other subjects, developing teaching materials, identifying instructional resources, and training teachers to deliver nutrition education.

Job opportunities for dietitians in child nutrition programs affect dietitians from the lunchroom to the classroom. School-based health centers—rapidly growing models for the delivery of comprehensive primary health care in elementary, middle, and high schools—afford another opportunity for dietitians interested in working with children and adolescents.[17] There is also a growing need in these school-based centers for dietitians certified by CDR for weight management of children and adolescents.[18]

Colleges and Universities

There are teaching opportunities for dietitians in culinary institutes, technical schools, and 2- or 4-year colleges. Such positions are often associated with programs for chefs, food service supervisors, dietetic technicians, dietary managers, entry-level dietitians, and hospitality managers. The emphasis is on teaching in the classroom, laboratory, or practice setting. Course responsibilities may include food preparation and food science, basic and applied nutrition, meal management, cultural food practices, food service management and equipment, nutrition assessment and therapy, nutrition counseling and education, and community nutrition.

University faculty roles are quite varied. In addition to their teaching responsibilities, university faculty are required to conduct research and provide service within the institution, community, or profession. They advise students on academic choices and research, serve on committees, consult with community groups, share their expertise with the media and the public, and provide departmental and university leadership for nutrition-related initiatives.

Higher education can include teaching other groups of students. For example, some institutions offer nutrition courses for nondietetics majors to fulfill requirements for general education, teacher certification, or health and physical education. Programs in the allied health professions may include nutrition courses. Dietitians can teach courses in nutritional anthropology or epidemiology, often included as part of the master's degree in public health programs.

Medical and Dental Education

Some graduate-trained dietitians are engaged in medical and dental education. Such a role requires assertiveness and creativity to convince administrators of the unique contributions that dietitians have to offer in medical and dental education.[19] For an emphasis on prevention and health promotion, nutrition is a required component and dietitians are unquestionably the best-qualified persons to provide this education. An in-depth knowledge of nutrition science and medical nutrition therapy is required. Additionally, medical and dental nutrition educators must possess leadership ability, self-direction, strong communication skills, conceptual thinking skills, time management techniques, and flexibility.

Nutrition education can occur at any level of a medical or dental curriculum. It may consist of nutrition science with clinical application during the first 2 years while basic information is the major part of the curriculum. As students enter the clinical part of their program, sample meals featuring special diets are often effective teaching tools. Nutrition rounds and seminars can be incorporated when students are in residencies. Practicing dietitians can be involved in problem-based learning as an effective way to make nutrition relevant for future medical practice.[20]

Nursing and Allied Health Nutrition Education

Nutrition services are often provided by nondietitians, depending on the practice setting and contributions of various health professionals. For example, nurses regularly monitor food intake, evaluate laboratory values indicative of nutritional status, and give patients nutritional advice.[21] Dental hygienists and health educators often screen for health or nutritional problems and provide education and intervention. All health professionals should understand the role nutrition plays in wellness and disease prevention, and they need training on appropriate interventions. It is generally agreed that nutrition education for nurses and other health professionals should be increased.

The ADA supports nutrition education for the health professions and advocates for the inclusion of nutrition in didactic, clinical, and continuing education programs. Dietitians are prepared to provide leadership for such programs and to direct nutrition education efforts in schools of medicine, nursing, pharmacy, allied health, social work, and occupational and physical therapy. However, there is a shortage of qualified faculty in this area.

Industry-Based Education

Companies that manufacture medical nutrition products often employ dietitians to provide technical and clinical information to the sales force and to other personnel, including clinicians, retail pharmacists, and educators of healthcare professionals. Dietitians may educate via telephone, written correspondence, electronic mail, and by personal visits. They may organize educational conferences and disseminate proceedings. They may participate in developing video, audio, and slide programs; technical monographs; newsletters; brochures; and professional and patient education publications on topics of medical nutrition therapy.

Companies that manufacture institutional equipment, food products, supplemental products such as high-protein and other preparations for tube feedings, infant formula, and supplements for nutritional additives, may also employ dietitians to help promote and demonstrate the use of the products.

Personal characteristics and skills necessary for success in industry-based education include technical and professional proficiency, ability to critically and objectively analyze issues, attention to detail, high work standards, skill in written and oral communications, adaptability, and ability to tolerate stress. Clearly, such positions require a proficiency in nutritional sciences, practitioner experience, conceptual and analytic skills, altruistic values, and a service ethic.

Worksite Nutrition Education

As increased attention is given to the role of nutrition in health and disease prevention, more opportunities for dietitians will open in worksite wellness programs. These worksites may include manufacturing plants, insurance companies, or service organizations. Some of these positions will focus entirely on nutrition education and may include screening for nutritional risk, program development, leading classes and demonstrations, creating exhibits and displays, and evaluating the effectiveness of nutrition education initiatives. Dietitians in these positions may provide valuable experience for dietetic interns or other students as well.

Worksite education opportunities can also include coordinators of training in large dietetics departments or at the regional level of contract food and nutrition service companies. Dietitians in such roles may oversee a dietetic internship, coordinate in-service training for food service and other personnel, and direct training for students from affiliating programs. Individuals with the appropriate background may be promoted to director of training and development at the institutional or corporate level.

The Dietitian in Research

Much of the research in nutrition and dietetics is conducted by students and faculty in colleges and universities. Some of these researchers are Registered Dietitians; others are food or nutrition scientists. Most faculty members conduct research as well as teach as part of their responsibilities. They may conduct laboratory research such as metabolic studies in human nutrient requirements or in food science to determine the utilization of specific food components. Other studies may be conducted in controlled working environments, as, for example, food service management productivity studies. Other types of research may deal with applied studies in nutrition education and data collection through surveys.

In clinical studies, dietitians may be part of a research team where knowledge of foods and diets is critical. Dietitians function to collect dietary and anthropometric data, teach nutrition protocols to participants, oversee food preparation in the metabolic kitchen, and work with team members.

Further career opportunities for dietitians in research are described in Chapter 13.

Career Preparation

Interest in research can develop early. Fundamental skill development often begins with an undergraduate research course, completion of an honors research study, or summer work in a research laboratory. One or more years practicing in a hospital, nursing home, clinic, or community setting is the first step toward success for a dietitian in education or research. First-hand experience leads to a valuable understanding of the practice milieu and the ability to draw from these backgrounds for illustrations and examples.

Most dietitians in education and research have attained at least a master's degree, and many have earned a doctorate. In addition, these individuals tend to be creative, intellectually curious, and self-directed achievers. They love libraries and they enjoy working at a scholarly level. Because much of their work involves communication and motivating others, they also must have good interpersonal skills.

Education and Research Practice Groups

Dietitians in education and research have numerous opportunities to unite with colleagues having similar interests (Table 10-3). As noted earlier, the ADA practice groups promote networking, mentoring, information exchange, professional enhancement, and leadership opportunities in organized areas of practice. Generally practice groups offer their members continuing education programs, quarterly newsletters, forums for exploring practice issues, and innovative products and services.

Table 10-3. Purpose of ADA Practice Groups for Dietitians in Research and Education

Nutrition Research Practice Group
   Promotes visibility of nutrition research and communication between researchers and practitioners.
Dietetic Educators of Practitioners
   Unites members of the ADA who are interested in or engaged in educating dietitians and dietetic technicians; represents the concerns of dietetic educators to the ADA, the government, institutions of higher learning, and the public.
Nutrition Educators of Health Professionals
   Advocates improvement in the quality of nutrition education of medical, dental, nursing, and allied health students; provides a forum for communication and information exchange between members, especially new educators; offers expertise in the development of nutrition curricula for undergraduate and graduate education.
Nutrition Education for the Public
   Champions improved well-being of the public by providing leadership in nutrition education planning, implementation, and evaluation; provides members with resources and opportunities to enhance both personal skills and nutrition expertise.

Source: Adapted with permission from *Dietetics Practice Group Information.* American Dietetic Association.

SUMMARY

Both education and research are essential for advancement of the dietetics profession. To prepare for these careers, students are encouraged to become associate members of the ADA, join relevant ADA practice groups, seek career advice or mentoring from dietitians in education and research, enroll in pertinent elective courses, and begin planning for graduate study.

Dietitians with expertise in worksite wellness, sports and cardiovascular nutrition, and disordered eating are increasingly in demand in nontraditional settings. They must be creative and adept in the promotion of healthy eating behaviors. In addition, nutrition education must be presented in a manner that is directly usable by consumers. The dietitian must also be able to translate scientific information into "user-friendly" terms.

DEFINITIONS

Academic Health Centers. Hospitals, medical centers, or clinics affiliated with a medical school or medical residency program.

Anorexia Nervosa. An eating disorder in which preoccupation with dieting and thinness leads to excessive weight loss.

Bulimia Nervosa. An eating disorder involving frequent episodes of binge eating and nearly always followed by purging.

Cardiovascular Nutrition. Application of medical nutrition therapy for those with heart and blood vessel conditions or to prevent the diseases.

Disordered Eating. Abnormal eating patterns.

Health Promotion. Education and preventive measures directed toward basically healthy populations to foster wellness.

Networking. Activities directed toward making connections with others through varied contacts.

Nontraditional Job. Job or position outside the usual or most common areas of practice.

Sports Nutrition. The area of nutrition specific to the needs of those who participate in sports activities.

Value System. Set of principles guiding actions that adhere to professional and ethical practice.

Wellness. State of optimal health and the absence of disease.

REFERENCES

1. Simopoulos, A. "Declaration of Olympia on Nutrition and Fitness." *Nutr Today* 3(1996): 250–252.
2. American Dietetic Association. Compensation and Benefits Survey of the Dietetics Profession 2009. www.eatright.org. Accessed October 5, 2009.
3. "Trends in the United States: Consumer Attitudes and the Supermarket." 2000. Food Marketing Institute: Washington, D.C. www.fmi.org (Accessed April 27, 2009).
4. Kapica, C. J.O.S. Maillet. "A Business Rotation for Dietitians—An Imperative in the New Millennium." *J Am Diet Assoc* 102(2002): 1220.
5. Indorato, D.A. "Innovative Services by and for Dietitians." *Today's Dietitian* 3, no. 4(2001): 16–19.
6. Finn, S.C. "The Dietitian in Business and Communications." In *Dietetics Practice and Future Trends.* E.A. Winterfeldt, M. Bogle, L.L. Ebro. Aspen Publishers: Gaithersburg, MD; 1998, p. 250.
7. Pangan, T. and C. Bedner. "Dietitian Business Websites: A Survey of Their Profitability and How You Can Make Yours Profitable." *J Am Diet Assoc* 101, no. 4(2002): 399–402.
8. Golson, S.K. "Make Time for Daily Physical Activity." *J Am Diet Assoc* 109, no. 1(2009): 18.

9. CDC. "Deaths: Final Data for 2005." National Center for Health Statistics. www.cdc.gov (Accessed February 10, 2009).

10. CDC. "Overweight Among Children and Adolescents, 16–19 Years of Age, by Selected Characteristics. U.S 1963–65 through 2005–2006." www.cdc.gov (Accessed April 28, 2009).

11. ADA. "Position of the American Dietetic Association: Dietitians of Canada and the American College of Sports Medicine: Nutrition and Athletic Performance." *J Am Diet Assoc* 100, no. 12(2000): 1543–1556.

12. Clark, N. "Identifying the Educational Needs of Aspiring Sports Nutritionists." *J Am Diet Assoc* 100, no. 12(2000): 1522–1524.

13. Shattuck, D. "Sports Nutritionists Feel the Competitive Edge." *J Am Diet Assoc* 101, no. 5(2001): 517–518.

14. Evans, W.J. and D. Cyr-Campbell. "Nutrition, Exercise, and Healthy Aging." *J Am Diet Assoc* 97(1997): 632–638.

15. Seymour, M., S.L. Hoerr, and Y. L. Huang. "Inappropriate Dieting Behavior and Related Lifestyle Factors in Young Adults: Are College Students Different?" *J Am Nutr Educ* 29(1997): 21–26.

16. Ammerman, S.D., G.H. Shih, and J. Ammerman. "Unique Considerations for Treating Eating Disorders in Adolescents and Preventive Interventions." *Topics in Clin Nutr* 12(1996): 79–85.

17. Juszcak, L., M. Fisher, J.C. Lear, and S.B. Friedman. "Back to School: Training Opportunities in School-Based Health Centers." *J Dev Behav Pediatr* 16(1995): 101–104.

18. ADA. "Certificate of Training in Childhood and Adolescent Weight Management." www.eatright.org (Accessed September 10, 2009).

19. Kolasa, K.M. and A.B. Lasswell. "Dietitians as Medical Educators." *Topics in Clin Nutr* 10(1995): 20–28.

20. Reiter, S.A., D.N. Rasmann-Nuhlicek, K. Biernat, and S.L. Lawrence. "Registered Dietitians as Problem-Based Learning Facilitators in a Nutrition Curriculum for Freshman Medical Students." *J Am Diet Assoc* 94(1994): 652–654.

21. Weigley, E.S. "Nutrition in Nursing Education and Beginning Practice." *J Am Diet Assoc* 94(1994): 654–656.

Part IV

Roles Essential for Dietitians

CHAPTER 11

The Dietitian as Manager and Leader

"Skills such as team building, delegation, communication, negotiation, and self-management are fundamental to high performance. Fortunately, these can be learned and enhanced through continuing education and training."[1]

OUTLINE

- Introduction
- Management and Leadership
- Leadership
  - Attaining Leadership Skills
  - Developing Leadership Talent
  - Leadership for Quality and Efficiency
- Management Functions
- Skills and Abilities of Managers
  - Human Relations Skills
  - Technical Skills
  - Conceptual Skills
  - Common Competencies for Healthcare Managers
- Further Management Roles
- Summary

INTRODUCTION

Management is often thought of as the responsibilities and challenges that have to do with "being in charge" or being "the boss" of a department, and therefore, the entry-level dietitian often believes that he or she does not need to be concerned with knowing how to manage. In reality, all dietitians, regardless of their job title or job responsibilities, perform many managerial functions and need to develop managerial skills. The clinical dietitian, the food service manager, the nutritionist in community nutrition programs, the educator, the private practitioner, the dietitian in business and industry, and healthcare administration all perform management functions. Among these functions are setting goals, managing resources, integrating and coordinating personnel activities, training personnel and allied professionals, communicating, and promoting quality control.

Ten so-called "soft skills" are necessary hallmarks of successful managers. They include a strong work ethic, a positive attitude, great communication skills, time management abilities, teamwork, self-confidence, ability to accept and learn from criticism, flexibility, adaptability, and the ability to work under pressure. All dietitians need to develop these skills regardless of their particular area of practice.[2] In this chapter, we discuss

Table 11-1. Balancing Management and Leadership

The Focus on Management	The Vision of Leadership
Do things right	Do the right things
Direct operations	Monitor guest expectations
Enforce policies and rules	Communicate vision and values
Design procedures and tasks	Manage systems and processes
Control results	Support people
Foster stability	Engage in continuous improvement

Source: Woods, R.H. and J.Z. King. *Quality Leadership and Management in the Hospitality Industry.* Educational Institute of the American Hotel and Motel Association: East Lansing, MI; 1996, p. 20.

management and leadership functions and skills and how each relates to professional practice in dietetics.

MANAGEMENT AND LEADERSHIP

Management and leadership have many overlapping characteristics, but they are not the same. According to Peter Drucker,[3] known as the "father of modern management," management is doing things right, while leadership is doing the right things. The manager makes things happen and will use many leadership activities in doing so. Some skills, however, are unique to the leader. In Table 11-1, several activities are illustrated that balance management and leadership.

LEADERSHIP

Drucker[4] points out that leadership is a means to an end—not just a quality to be desired. He considers the three most important characteristics for successful leadership to be:

1. Thinking through the organization's mission, defining it, and establishing it clearly and visibly. The leader sets the goals and priorities, and maintains the standards.
2. Viewing leadership as a responsibility and not a rank or privilege. Effective leaders are rarely permissive, but when things go wrong, they do not blame others. They encourage and help develop strong associates and subordinates.
3. Earning trust in order to have followers. To trust a leader, it is not necessary to like or to agree, rather trust is the conviction that the leader means what he or she says and has integrity.

Schroeder,[5] a successful dietitian-leader, believes that integrity and vision are hallmarks of leadership success.

Several theories of leadership and leadership styles are discussed in the book *Leadership in Dietetics*.[6] All dietitians will benefit from the examples of leadership in action outlined in this book.

Attaining Leadership Skills

A question often debated is whether people are born leaders or whether they develop leadership skills and thereby become leaders. In support of the view that leadership skills can be acquired, several actions that make for leadership development are the following:[7]

- Be creative by encouraging innovative staff performance, involving coworkers in decision making, and rewarding them for contributions.
- Form teams that will foster employee satisfaction, personal mastery, empowerment, and effective problem solving.
- Take risks by showing that it is acceptable to try nontraditional methods, thereby fostering ingenuity and resourcefulness.
- Expect failure and state this to employees so they know that creativity cannot be hampered by fear of failure.
- Encourage continuous learning so that higher levels of competence and responsibility can be achieved.
- Communicate effectively to promote trust and high performance within teams.
- Symbolize the unit's activities by demonstrating knowledge of "how things work."
- Benchmark by comparing performance with that of other operators and finding better methods and systems through sharing information with colleagues. This will provide further ideas for planning.
- Walk around, be visible, and be involved with the daily activities of the unit.

Developing Leadership Talent

A research study by Cleveland[8] indicates that the highest performing leaders have characteristic integrity, honesty, and personal capabilities such as innovation and self-development. In addition, they focus on results, champion change, and inspire others to higher performance. To develop leadership talent in healthcare organizations, it is essential to identify key leader competencies; develop effective job design; focus on leadership recruitment, development, and retention; and provide leadership training and development in all levels of the organization through ongoing leadership assessment and performance management. Leadership training, development, and performance management are effective when incorporated into the real-work environment of the leader.

Leadership for Quality and Efficiency

Leadership development programs, increasingly conducted in hospitals and other healthcare organizations, improve both the quality and efficiency of care. Opportunities found to result from three qualitative studies of leadership development are the following:[9]

- Increase the caliber of the workforce.
- Enhance efficiency in the organization's education and development activities.
- Reduce turnover and related expenses.
- Focus organizational attention on specific priorities.

Potential activities to improve leadership development are shown in Table 11-2.

Table 11-2. Using Leadership Development to Improve Quality

Opportunities for Leadership Development	Potential Activities
Improve caliber and quality of workforce.	1. Improve overall leadership skills of workforce to increase competencies and capabilities of employees. 2. Focus training in specific areas related to cost reduction, quality of care, etc. 3. Provide training and development in focused areas. 4. Create opportunities for application of new skills, including follow-up after developmental programs.
Improve efficiency in organizational education and development.	1. Focus development agenda for employees to reduce duplication and enable cross-communication in employee education and training activities. 2. Take advantage of opportunities to provide development training and education in-house to reduce travel expense and extend reach of programs.

(continues)

Table 11-2. Using Leadership Development to Improve Quality
(*continued*)

Opportunities for Leadership Development	Potential Activities
Reduce employee turnover and related expenses.	1. Tie leadership activities to employee satisfaction surveys to emphasize importance of employee retention and satisfaction.
	2. Provide focused training for clinically trained persons to learn leadership skills to reduce employee frustration and improve likelihood of success.
Focus organizational attention on strategic priorities.	1. Deliver leadership development training and education linked to the organization's strategic planning process.
	2. Design and deliver specific education and development modules, courses, and programs focused on quality of care and operational efficiency.
	3. Tie performance evaluation metrics to organizational goals, such as improving quality of care, reducing costs, improving patient satisfaction, holding leaders accountable for success while making appropriate education and training available to help people meet goals.

Source: Adapted from McAlearney, A.S. "Using Leadership Development Programs to Improve Quality and Efficiency in Healthcare." *J Healthcare Management* 53, no. 5(2008): 319–331.

MANAGEMENT FUNCTIONS

Management is usually defined in terms of the traditional functions described by management experts. Although the number of functions may vary according to the way in which they are presented, the following six are universally accepted.[10] It should be noted these are essentially advanced management skills needed by the food service professional in administrative areas of practice.

1. Planning is the activity of setting goals and objectives. The extent of the planning, from setting broad, long-range goals for a large organization to planning of shorter-term goals, will usually be determined by where persons are in the organizational hierarchy.

2. Organizing is the reflection of how the organization accomplishes its goals and objectives. The tasks to be performed, assignment of tasks, allocation of resources, and flow of authority and communication are established.
3. Coordinating involves activities that lead to the efficient use of resources to attain the goals and objectives.
4. Staffing means determining human resource needs, then recruiting, selecting, hiring, and training the necessary staff.
5. Directing (or leading) refers to those activities that enable accomplishment of the organization goals, communicate those goals, and create an atmosphere that encourages commitment and desired performance.
6. Controlling occurs when performance is assessed against standards that have been translated from the goals and objectives and corrective measures are applied as needed.

Crucial activities characteristic of the successful leader in terms of management roles are shown in Table 11-3.

Table 11-3. Thirty Crucial Activities for the Successful Leader

Role Set	Mintzberg's (1980) 10 Managerial Roles	30 Crucial Activities
Motivating others	Figurehead Liaison Leader	1. Recruiting professionals 2. Making decisions regarding professionals and managerial salaries 3. Devising work procedures for professionals 4. Devising work procedures for nonprofessionals 5. Promoting and rewarding professionals and managers 6. Conducting employee and management development and training 7. Disciplining professional and managerial employees 8. Motivating and directing immediate subordinates 9. Dealing with personal and interpersonal problems

(continues)

Table 11-3. Thirty Crucial Activities for the Successful Leader *(continued)*

Role Set	Mintzberg's (1980) 10 Managerial Roles	30 Crucial Activities
Scanning the environment	Monitor Disseminator	10. Market research 11. Product research 12. Long-range planning 13. Criteria systems development to control quality 14. Decisions regarding financial and management information systems
Negotiating the political terrain	Spokesperson Negotiator Disturbance handler	15. Conducting public relations 16. Lobbying 17. Conducting labor negotiations 18. Establishing agreements with other institutions 19. Negotiating with powerful external organizations 20. Creating and changing professional job unity 21. Making decisions regarding changes in decision-making and authority structure 22. Influencing decisions of administration or the board 23. Influencing decisions made by the medical staff 24. Arbitrating between internal units and/or other departments
Generating and allocating resources	Entrepreneur Resource allocator	25. Decisions regarding buying procedure 26. Decisions regarding working capital expenses 27. Decisions regarding maintaining building and equipment 28. Decisions regarding charges and prices for services 29. Decisions regarding new construction 30. Decisions regarding general operation

Source: Jackson, R. *Nutrition and Food Services for Integrated Health Care: A Handbook for Leaders.* Aspen Publishers: Gaithersburg, MD; 1997, p. 74.

SKILLS AND ABILITIES OF MANAGERS

Three fundamental cross sections of skills needed by managers to function effectively are: human relations, technical, and conceptual (Figure 11-1).

Earlier traditional views of management held that top managers primarily needed human relations and conceptual skills, while the more contemporary view is that technical skills are increasingly important for the top manager, especially in small organizations and in those with flattened and decentralized organizational patterns. Middle managers require an almost equal distribution of skills among the three types, while the supervisor is viewed as needing slightly more conceptual skills. In the contemporary view, supervisors and employees in the organization also need a share of all of the skills, but the emphasis is on the technical. The use of particular skills will vary from day to day with changes in the work environment such as the need to hire and train new employees or to engage in long-range strategic planning. The three skill areas are discussed in the following sections.

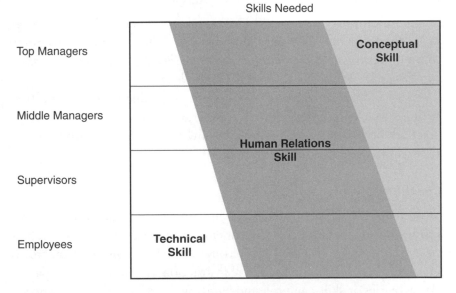

FIGURE 11-1. Contemporary Cross Section of Management Skills.

Source: Woods, R.H. and J.Z. King. *Quality Leadership and Management in the Hospitality Industry.* Educational Institute of the American Hotel and Motel Association: East Lansing, MI; 1996, p. 16.

Human Relations Skills

Interpersonal Relationships

Interpersonal skills are always rated highly when management skills are described or studied. The ability to work with others toward common goals is the number one factor denoting success among healthcare multidepartmental managers.[11] Numerous books and articles have been published about establishing and maintaining interpersonal relationships. Every dietitian will benefit from including one or more in his or her library. The *Harvard Business Review* is also an excellent source for readings in this area.

Generational diversity, or the involvement of several distinct generations in the workplace, presents another aspect of achieving successful working relationships.[12] Different generations of workers are assumed to have different loyalties and expectations resulting in the need for open-mindedness, effective communication, and respect for others on the part of the manager.

Communications

Communication at both an organizational and a personal level is an essential part of every manager's job. Two excellent references concerning communications are *Communicating as Professionals*[13] and *Communication and Education Skills: The Dietitian's Guide.*[14]

Verbal and nonverbal skills as well as listening skills are vital in practice. Because communicating online has become so important in all area of practice, dietitians need to be aware of how to fully and effectively create, access, share, and use online information.

Coaching and Mentoring

Most dietitians will be, at some time in their career, in the position of assisting and supporting a coworker or employee as they learn a new job or develop new skills, and thus will become a coach or mentor. A mentor is a person who teaches through verbal instruction, demonstration of particular activities or skills, and role-modeling, while the coach is one who inspires and motivates.[15] The successful dietitian in a work unit may function in either of these roles in order to accomplish needed tasks. Staff personnel perform at different levels and learn in different ways. It is the enterprising coach or mentor who is able to adapt actions to motivate, encourage, and support staff, thereby creating a productive and harmonious team. Mentoring is discussed in greater detail in Chapter 12.

Managing Conflict

Conflict occurs in any organization and may result from competition for resources, overlapping responsibilities, status struggles, poor communications, inadequate training, or differences in values and beliefs. The dietitian who recognizes causes of conflict and assists in taking steps to overcome the differences will be looked to as a manager and leader.

Networking

Networking within an organization leads to interconnectedness. People form networks for sharing social and business information and to increase professional competence. The manager or leader will seek opportunities to network and will further encourage others in the work unit to also network. Networking with other professionals through the dietetic practice groups of the ADA and other groups can lead to personal growth, a greater understanding of practice requirements, and enhanced performance in every area of practice.

Technical Skills

Technical skills are those that require a specialized knowledge of techniques, methods, procedures, and processes that accomplish the work of an organization. Several types are discussed.

Job Skills

The manager or leader has knowledge of what is required to perform in an organization, but may not actually perform the work except on an "as-needed" basis. However, this knowledge allows the manager to supervise those with the specific skills to fulfill the job requirements. The need to have job "know-how" is essential to assess performance, meet goals, and ensure quality outputs.

Resource Management

Financial management, including cost controls, comes to mind first when the management of resources is described as a management function.

Resources, however, can also mean job-related supplies and equipment, staff assistance, and even time and energy. Every dietitian and dietetic technician carries certain responsibilities for managing resources and also may be involved in budgeting and long-range planning.

The importance of teaching financial management in dietetics programs is emphasized by dietetics program directors. In one survey, educators agreed or strongly agreed with the statement: "Entry-level Registered Dietitians need to be trained in financial management concepts as well as clinical concepts in order to be competent practitioners."[16]

Benchmarking is a process that measures the efficiency of work, the products produced, and the services for comparison and improvement.[17] This process is used in both health care and food services. Performance measures that include financial management, customer service, human resources, and operational activities are evaluated in the benchmarking process. Measurements used provide information that can be compared and used for improvement.

Training and Staff Development

The responsibility for hiring and training a workforce is primarily that of upper-level management, however, all professionals will at times help train and develop new employees or other professionals. The team concept often followed in healthcare institutions, food service, and hospitality requires that all members of a team function fully and efficiently. Further, team members must know their job-related roles as well as their expected roles as a team member. Efficiency evolves from knowledge and practice and must be encouraged and assisted by those already experienced within an organization.

Technology Know-How

The importance of communication has been discussed as a human relations skill. Knowing how to access and use all available technology for communication is a must for all professionals in the modern workplace. Online information is rapidly becoming the means by which professionals remain current. Conferences, workshops, meetings, and classes are offered by teleconference, online, or by similar means using newer technology.

Not only is communications technology of increasing importance, but technology related to better and faster job performance benefits both individuals and an organization. To the extent that professionals become experts in the technology needed for their jobs, they will also become mentors and coaches for others.

Technology is increasingly used in food production and food service. Examples are used for developing work schedules, purchasing and inventory control, keeping employee records, and establishing production schedules. These activities point to the need for continued training and staff development.

Team Building

A team functions in ways that support individual efforts and lead to greater productivity. Teams vary in number, may be formal or informal, and may form in a variety of ways. For instance, a team may be formed within a department or from several departments or disciplines to accomplish more than can be accomplished by individuals. Teams may also be temporary or permanent.

The value of teams lies in sharing knowledge and working toward common goals using the experience and expertise of several in decision making and problem solving. The manager or leader encourages teams and helps make them effective by arranging for persons to participate and providing for training of team members as needed. Teams function best when they are empowered with authority or legal power to reach a level of self-management.[18]

Work groups are often formed of persons working together for a common purpose. As with teams, they may be formally constituted or may function in a more informal way such as a gathering of people to solve daily problems. The group leader has several tasks, which include understanding the internal workings of the group, planning ahead and being proactive, and managing interpersonal relations for group cohesion.

Quality Management

Quality is a term defined as meeting standards and expectations, sometimes in terms of high quality or above a norm or average. The Quality Management Committee of the ADA provides direction for monitoring, developing, approving, evaluating, and maintaining quality management in dietetics. The ten members of the group interact with the scope of practice framework committee, the evidence-based practice committee, and the nutrition care process committee. Quality assurance in practice results through the coordinated efforts of these groups.

Dietitians in all areas of practice can monitor their own quality of work through the Code of Ethics, the Standards of Professional Performance, and the Professional Development Portfolio. The outcome is competent practice and a basis for quality improvement as indicated.

Every institution, department, business, or professional association strives to produce quality goods, services, or people. Rather than relying on subjective methods to detect quality, most organizations establish performance measures by which they assess and ensure continuous quality.

In dietetics, performance standards are in effect and are described in other sections of this book. Food production managers use performance measures to ensure the quality of the food service. Patient satisfaction surveys are used for ongoing assessment of the services received. Clinical outcomes can be measured for quality through specific established indicators. The community nutritionist measures quality of service by satisfactory outcomes of persons receiving instruction and care. The educator measures outcomes and the quality of the education by how his or her students perform.

Even though "quality" is a somewhat elusive descriptor, it is part of every dietitian's job responsibility and is a managerial function.

Conceptual Skills

The manager or leader performs a certain number of activities based on thinking about the bigger picture beyond the technical aspects of his or her position. The ability to visualize the future, to plan and set goals, to provide direction in an organization, and to model professional behavior constitutes conceptual ability or skill.

Strategic Planning and Goal Setting

In general, strategic planning occurs at the upper levels of management because it requires data gathering and analysis; development of strategies, goals, and objectives, and implementation of action plans. All professionals, however, at all levels in an organization participate in data gathering and in setting short- and long-term goals. They are a part of the planning process to set direction and plans of action for the organization.

Some plans are general, such as the determination of values, mission, and vision statements.[19] Others are more detailed and may be developed at the supervisory level. If operational plans are short range, they are usually expected to occur within a year. Long-term plans extend beyond a year and up to 10 years. The food and nutrition professional often contributes to both types of planning by conducting feasibility studies, cost-effectiveness studies, and quality-control measures.

Ethical Conduct

In dietetics the *Code of Ethics for the Profession of Dietetics*[20] is the guiding document to ethical practice. In any institution, the manager or leader assists in developing organization practices and policies that promote ethical practice. Such practices are established in purchasing, financial management, patient care issues, and information provided by patients and clients. The manager or leader sets the example for ethical behavior and integrity built on openness and trust.

Managing Change

Change occurs when there is dissatisfaction with events as they are and a desire to change them. Change may occur slowly or rapidly as in the event of sudden or unplanned circumstances. The leader who welcomes change and uses it to motivate and improve a department or unit's functions will be the most successful. When members of a unit work together to make changes, the efforts are usually rewarded by acceptance of the new procedure by all those affected. In contrast, if change is imposed by the leader without input from the other members, there is often resistance and slow acceptance.

Dietitians who counsel clients to make changes do not always meet with success. Time constraints and client expectations and motivations that differ from those of the dietitian are factors in the change process. Change models that take into consideration the complexities of behavior and one's approach to what it takes to help people change are often helpful. One approach is the use of goal setting in a way that the client being counseled is a part of the process and understands the expected outcome.[21]

The first step to recognition of the need for change is identifying the problem. One or more achievable goals for overcoming the problem are set in the second step of the process, followed by actions toward achieving the goals. In the action step, persons typically mobilize their personal and social resources and identify barriers to reaching the goal. Self-monitoring and reward provide additional motivation to successfully attain the goal. The reward may be external, but a very effective reward is the internal one such as learning that leads to sustained performance and further goal setting.

Dietetics professionals constantly face change because of new developments in health care, organizational changes, and shifts in management with new mission and vision goals. Even environmental and political situations create change. When changes are viewed as opportunities, they are more likely to lead to positive results. The creative manager or leader helps create an atmosphere that welcomes and plans for this outcome.

Common Competencies for Healthcare Managers

The Healthcare Leadership Alliance is a consortium of six major professional organizations.[22] A research study conducted by the Alliance reported on five competencies common among practicing healthcare managers (Figure 11-2).

1. Communication and relationship management: The ability to communicate clearly and concisely with internal and external customers and to facilitate interactions with individuals and groups.

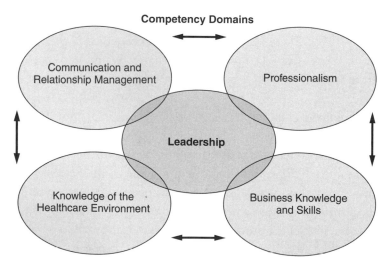

FIGURE 11-2. The Healthcare Leadership Alliance Competency Model

Source: Stefl, M.E. "Common Competencies for All Healthcare Managers: The Healthcare Leadership Alliance Model." *J Healthcare Management* 53, no. 6(2008): 360–373.

2. Leadership: The ability to inspire excellence, to create and attain shared vision, and to manage change.
3. Professionalism: The ability to align personal and organizational conduct with ethical and professional standards that include a responsibility to the patient and community, a service orientation, and a commitment to lifelong learning and improvement.
4. Knowledge of the healthcare environment: The demonstrated understanding of the healthcare system, and the environment in which healthcare managers and providers function.
5. Business skills and knowledge: The ability to apply business principles, including systems thinking, in the healthcare environment.

Table 11-4. Mintzberg's 10 Managerial Roles

Managerial Role	Behavior
Interpersonal	
Figurehead	Represents the organization on formal ceremonial occasions
Liaison	Interacts with peers in the organization, other colleagues, and people outside the vertical chain of command to gain favors and gather information
Leader	Motivates and guides staff
Informational	
Monitor	Scans the environment for information, asks for information from subordinates and peers, and receives unsolicited information
Disseminator	Transmits information into the organization
Spokesperson	Sends information into the external environment
Decisional	
Entrepreneur	Initiates change to improve the unit and to adapt to a changing environment
Disturbance handler	Takes charge when the organization is threatened and when there is conflict and pressure beyond the manager's control
Resource allocator	Decides where the organization will expend its efforts
Negotiator	Deals with situations in which the manager feels compelled to enter negotiations on behalf of the organization

Source: Barker, A.N., M.B.F. Arensberg, and M.R. Schiller. *Leadership in Dietetics: Achieving a Vision for the Future.* The American Dietetic Association: Chicago; 1994, p. 55.

FURTHER MANAGEMENT ROLES

A noted management expert and author, Mintzberg,[23] describes a manager's job in terms of roles and behaviors. The three categories are: interpersonal, informational, and decisional (Table 11-4). The roles overlap and may gain in importance depending on the content and purposes of the manager's work. Interpersonal roles are a part of the formal authority of the manager and because of many interpersonal interactions, the informational role is critical. By using the information gathered from the interpersonal and informational roles, the manager is central in making decisions for the organizational unit.

SUMMARY

Managers and leaders possess many characteristics that are similar, but there are differences in roles and responsibilities. The skillful manager possesses human, technical, and conceptual abilities that permit him or her to accomplish work through coworkers and to attain goals. The leader may perform some or all of these same functions but will also inspire, motivate, and create a sense of unity and purpose. The dietitian, regardless of the area of practice, must perform managerial functions such as goal setting, communicating, team building, and managing resources. Many critical functions in the workplace will also require the dietitian to lead.

DEFINITIONS

Benchmarking. Comparing performance measures for the development of better methods and procedures.

Coaching. The process by which a teacher or guide inspires and motivates.

Leadership. The qualities that allow an individual to influence the actions of others.

Management. The activities by which an organization functions.

Mentoring. Teaching and guiding by instructing, demonstrating, encouraging, and role-modeling.

Resource Management. The handling of money, equipment and supplies, or personnel essential to the administration of an organizational unit.

Strategic Planning. Long-range planning that involves data gathering, data analysis, development of goals and objectives, and action plans.

REFERENCES

1. Covey, S.R. *Principle-Centered Leadership.* Simon and Schuster: New York; 1990, p. 184.
2. Gould, R.S. and D. Canter. "Management Matters." *J Am Diet Assoc* 108, no. 11(2008): 1834–1836.
3. Drucker, P.F. *Managing for the Future: The 1990s and Beyond.* Ruman Talley Books/Plume: New York; 1992.
4. Jackson, R. *Nutrition and Food Services for Integrated Health Care: A Handbook for Leaders.* Aspen Publishers: Gaithersburg, MD; 1997, p. 65.
5. Weisberg, K. "Spirited Pioneer." *Foodservice Director.* May (2007): 65–66.
6. Barker, A.N., M.B.F. Arensberg, and M.R. Schiller. *Leadership in Dietetics: Achieving a Vision for the Future.* The American Dietetic Association: Chicago; 1994, pp. 60–65.
7. See Note 4, p. 92
8. Wells, W. and W. Hejna. "Developing Leadership Talent in Healthcare Organizations." *Healthcare Financial Management* 63, no. 1(2009): 66–69.
9. McAlearney, A.S. "Using Leadership Development Programs to Improve Quality and Efficiency in Healthcare." *J Healthcare Management* 53, no. 5(2008): 319–331.
10. See Note 2.
11. Carter, D.D. and M.F. Nettles. "Dietitians as Multidepartment Managers in Health Care Settings." *J Am Diet Assoc* 103, no. 2(2003): 237–240.
12. Brown, D. "Ways Dietitians of Different Generations Can Work Together." *J Am Diet Assoc* 103, no. 11(2003): 1461–1462.
13. Chernoff, R., ed. *Communicating as Professionals.* 2nd ed. The American Dietetic Association: Chicago; 1994, p. 26.
14. Holli, B.B. and R.J. Calabrese. *Communication and Education Skills: The Dietitian's Guide.* 2nd ed. Lea and Febiger: Philadelphia; 1991.
15. Hendricks, W., ed. *Coaching, Mentoring, and Managing.* Career Press: Franklin Lakes, NJ; 1996.
16. McKnight, L.E.G., M.L. Dundas, and J.T. Girvan. "Dietetics Program Directors Affirm the Importance of Teaching Financial Management Concepts in All Areas of Practice." *J Am Diet Assoc* 102, no. 2(2002): 82–84.
17. Johnson, B.C. and J. Chambers. "Foodservice Benchmarking: Practices, Attitudes, and Beliefs of Foodservice Directors." *J Am Diet Assoc* 100, no. 2(2000): 175–180.
18. See Note 5.
19. Spears, M. *Foodservice Organization: A Managerial and Systems Approach.* Prentice Hall: Englewood Cliffs, NJ; 1995, p. 108.

20. American Dietetic Association. "American Dietetic Association/Commission on Dietetic Registration Code of Ethics for the Profession of Dietetics and Process for Consideration of Ethics Issues." *J Am Diet Assoc* 109, no. 8(2009): 1461–1467.

21. Cullen, K.W., T. Baranowski, and S.P. Smith. "Using Goal Setting as a Strategy for Dietary Behavior Change." *J Am Diet Assoc* 101, no. 5(2001): 562–565.

22. Stefl, M.E. "Common Competencies for All Healthcare Managers: The Healthcare Leadership Alliance Model." *J of Healthcare Management* 53, no. 6(2008): 360–373.

23. See Note 5.

CHAPTER 12

The Dietitian as Educator

"Education is a lifelong process, an individual responsibility to be shared and used for personal growth and to benefit our customers and our community."[1]

OUTLINE

- Introduction
- Educational Activities
- Learning to Teach
  - Theories of Learning
  - Types of Learning
- Designing Instruction
  - Assessment of the Needs of Learners
  - Performance Objectives
  - Assessment Instruments
  - Instructional Strategy
  - Instructional Materials
  - Evaluation
  - Use of the Design
- Educator Roles
  - Mentor
  - Coach
  - Preceptor
  - Counselor
  - Communicator
- Types of Learning
  - Service Learning

· Problem-Based Learning
· Project-Based Learning
· Adults as Learners
· Teaching Groups and Teams
· Summary

INTRODUCTION

Dietitians sometimes reveal that they chose dietetics as a career in part because they did not view themselves as a teacher. The reality, however, is that all dietitians are educators, most frequently in locations other than the classroom. The educational settings are as diverse as the careers in which dietitians work; the learners are individuals and groups of all ages. For example, the dietitian who works in clinical dietetics in a hospital or other healthcare center teaches patients, families, and allied health personnel. A dietitian in food service management teaches and trains food service personnel and may teach personnel in other departments. Dietitians in business or private practice may teach patients, other personnel, and the public. In all areas of practice, the dietitian may also teach dietetic interns and dietetic technician students.

The educator role is one of the most important a dietitian fulfills. Knowledge of subject matter is attained by the professional through academic preparation in a degree program and practical experience in an internship. Added to this knowledge is an understanding of how to teach effectively and how people learn. Observation of other educators, continuing education, and professional experience as well as practice lead to expertise as an educator.

Dietitians need to possess several skills related to teaching. These include verbal and nonverbal communications, public speaking, behavior modification and motivation, principles of learning, teaching methods and techniques, and knowledge about how to work with groups. These skills can be learned and improved the more they are used.

EDUCATIONAL ACTIVITIES

The Commission on Dietetic Registration conducts periodic review of activities performed by Registered Dietitians and Dietetic Technicians, Registered. The following list of activities is typical of the educational activities that dietitians perform depending on each person's job requirements.[2]

1. *Nutrition education of public groups*
   Delivers preplanned educational programs
   Selects educational methodologies, develops materials, and delivers programs
   Establishes goals and priorities for educational programs
2. *Computer information systems*
   Uses computer technology to process data (e.g., nutrient analyses, patient/client information, production and purchasing records)
   Maintains effective communications among employees, clients, other professionals through e-mail and social networking
3. *Educational training*
   Trains employees and new professional staff
   Develops and presents seminars for health professionals and students
   Acts as a preceptor for dietetics and other students
   Teaches in educational institutions
   Plans, develops, and implements dietetics nutrition education courses for health professionals, students, and clients
4. *Nutrition education and counseling*
   Implements educational protocols and adapts as needed
   Assesses needs and evaluates effect of nutrition counseling
   Conducts group and individual educational sessions

LEARNING TO TEACH

The success of any educational undertaking is an outcome of the planning that occurs prior to the learning session. Many dietitians have taught inservice classes or community groups with inadequate time to plan and prepare or uncertainty about how to proceed, resulting in a disappointing session for all. Inexperience, lack of information about the learner and his or her background and needs, lack of knowledge about instructional methods, and inadequate preparation are factors that can lessen the effect of a learning situation.

The clinical dietitian who teaches patients will find it helpful to have an understanding of teaching skills as illustrated in Table 12-1. For instance, interpersonal skills help build trust and rapport between the patient and the dietitian. Essential teaching skills are general strategies that form a framework for most teaching. Adherence counseling skills help assess compliance to a treatment plan. Presentation skills help make instruction a learning experience; these skills improve the likelihood that learners will apply what they learn.[3]

Theories of Learning

Two major theories of learning, behavioral and cognitive, have been described.[4] Behaviorists concentrate on how individuals learn new habits or procedures through stimulus and response. Cognitive theorists believe that the learner becomes an active participant in the learning process and is goal-directed.

Table 12-1. Effective Patient Teaching Skills

Interpersonal Skills	Presentation Skills
Respect for the patient	Opening
Vocal behavior	Negotiating objectives
Body language	Organizational clarity
Essential Teaching Functions	Stimulus variety
Assessment	Highlighting
Evaluation	Active involvement
Feedback	Using visual aids
Independent practice	Use of examples
Adherence Counseling Skills	Closing
Specifying a behavioral plan	
Negotiating the treatment plan	
Accountability and follow-up	
Use of behavioral techniques	

Source: Roach, R.R., J.W. Pichert, B.A. Stetson, R.A. Lorenz, E.J. Boswell, and D.G. Schlundt. "Improving Dietitians' Teaching Skills." *J Am Diet Assoc* 92, no. 12(1992): 1466–1473.

Types of Learning

Education programs are based on learning outcomes, or categories of learning, described as domains of learning. One classification by Gagne describes five types of learning outcomes or skills as follows:[5]

1. Psychomotor skills: The learner acquires motor skills along with the know-how to perform tasks.
2. Intellectual skills: Information-processing skills allow the learner to perform a new activity.
3. Verbal processing skills: The learner is able to provide information through stating, listing, or describing something.
4. Attitudinal skills: The learner makes choices or decisions to act in certain ways. These may include long-term goals that determine a person's ability to perform psychomotor or other skills.
5. Cognitive skills: The learner has attained abstract strategies to become self-directed through the use of intellectual skills.

DESIGNING INSTRUCTION

The steps involved in preparing to teach are the following:

Assessment of the Needs of Learners

In this step, the instructor finds out what individuals already know and what they need to know. This may be accomplished through tests or surveys, oral interviews, or by focus groups and observation. At times, the need for instruction may result from a needs assessment, from practical experience with learning difficulties of earlier learners, by analysis of someone performing a job, or a change in organizational needs. It is important to know the present status of persons regarding their knowledge, skills, abilities, aptitudes, interests, personality, educational background, and psychological readiness to learn. It may not be possible to discern all these factors in every situation; however, this initial step is important to plan instruction to fit the learner's needs.

Performance Objectives

Based on the needs assessment, specific statements are written describing what the learner will be able to accomplish upon completion of the course.

The objectives identify the skills to be learned, the conditions under which they are performed, and the criteria for successful performance. The objectives need to be measurable and focused on the learner.[6]

A classification system for performance objectives often referenced by educators includes three categories or domains: cognitive, affective, and psychomotor. The cognitive domain includes the following six categories:[7]

1. Knowledge: Acquiring and remembering specific material.
2. Comprehension: Ability to grasp the meaning of the material.
3. Application: Ability to use learned material in new situations.
4. Analysis: Ability to break down material into its component parts for an understanding of how it is organized.
5. Synthesis: Ability to put parts together to form a new whole.
6. Evaluation: Ability to judge the value of material for a given purpose.

According to Bloom and colleagues,[8] learning progresses from the first or lowest level (knowledge) to the highest (evaluation).

The second, or affective, domain concerns changes in attitude, values, beliefs, appreciation, and interests. Krathwohl[9] and others have developed a listing of educational objectives in the affective domain. They are:

- Receiving: The learner becomes aware of and receives the lesson.
- Responding: The learner becomes involved in a subject or activity.
- Valuing: The learner believes in and accepts the value of the information.
- Organizing: The learner conceptualizes and organizes a value system.
- Characterizing: Values have been internalized and control behavior.

In the psychomotor domain, several levels are identified during which the development of manual or motor skills progresses to increasingly more difficult steps.[10]

1. Perception: The learner becomes aware of objects through the senses and selects the sensory perceptions needed to act.
2. Set: A readiness to perform tasks is demonstrated, both mentally and physically.
3. Guided response: The teacher or trainer guides the learner in an activity.

4. Mechanism: Through practice, the learner becomes proficient at the task.
5. Complex overt response: A level of skill is attained over time, or performance is characterized by accuracy and speed.
6. Adaptation/origination: Motor proficiency is altered in new situations and new physical acts based on skills attained are created or "originated."

A behavioral objective has three parts: a description of the skill or behavior identified in the analysis, a description of the conditions under which the learner carries out the task, and the criteria that will be used to evaluate learner performance.[11] An example of an objective demonstrating these parts follows:

• The clinical dietitian conducts a nutritional assessment for each patient admitted to the healthcare unit within 24 hours after admission and records the findings in the patient's chart.

The type of action is designated by the verb selected to demonstrate the action. Psychomotor skills are usually expressed in terms of an action verb, such as perform. Intellectual skills are shown by verbs such as discriminate, identify, classify, and demonstrate. Verbs that are general, such as know or understand, are too vague unless the specific behavior that demonstrates acquisition of knowledge can be described.

To decide if the objective is clear and feasible, the instructor constructs a test item to measure the learner's performance.

Assessment Instruments

The term assessment denotes broader activity than just testing and includes many types of activities that may be used to assess performance. When tests are used, the basic types are the pretest and the posttest. The pretest measures skills that have been identified as critical to beginning instruction and that the designer plans to develop in the instruction. If the material to be taught is new to the learner, a pretest is probably not necessary because it can be assumed that he or she has no background knowledge or skill in the subject. The posttest should focus on the objective. Its main purpose is to help the designer identify areas of instruction that need revision.

Several types of tests may be used, and the type is based on the objective. Examples of assessment instruments to measure performance, product, and attitudes include the following: a checklist, a rating scale that requires levels of discrimination (poor to excellent, for instance, the Likert scale), a frequency count, or a combination of formats.

Instructional Strategy

Instructional strategy refers to the sequencing and organizing of information to be learned and deciding on the delivery format. The objectives for lower-level skills are usually the starting point, progressing to higher levels of learning. Factors to be considered include: level of the learners, complexity of the material, type of learning to take place, activities to be included, and amount of time required to include all the events planned. Prior to actual instruction, it is helpful to consider the motivation of the learners. Motivation involves gaining the learners' attention by asking questions, creating mental challenges, using human interest examples, and humor. Establishing the relevancy of the material for the learners and instilling confidence that they can master the material are important.

The instructor next plans the format and presentation procedures for each objective or cluster of objectives. The learning activities may differ for the cognitive, affective, and psychomotor domains. In general, techniques used should actively involve the learner insofar as it is possible to do so.

The strengths and weaknesses of several teaching methods are shown in Table 12-2.

Job instruction training is a four-step process often used to teach skills. In the first step, the learner is prepared by putting him or her at ease, finding out what he or she already knows, stating the job to be learned, and developing interest. In step two, the material is presented and explained by stressing key points, instructing clearly and completely, illustrating and demonstrating, and then summarizing. Step three tests how much the learner has retained by practicing the procedure, coached by the trainer or instructor. The final step is to let the learner proceed with supervision to ensure the task is performed accurately and consistently.

Davis[12] describes ways to assist learners as they internalize new information:

1. Accept the fact that learners receive, think, and process information in different ways. The differences are most noticeable when the new

Table 12-2. Strengths and Weaknesses of Teaching Methods

Method	Strengths	Weaknesses

Lecture	Easy and efficient
	Conveys most information
	Reaches large numbers
	Minimum threat to learner
	Maximum control by
	    instructor
		Learner is passive
		Learning by listening
		Formal atmosphere
		May be dull, boring
		Not suited for higher-
		    level learning in
		    cognitive domain
		Not suited for
		    manual learning

Discussion
Panel
Debate
Case study
	More interesting, thus
	    motivating
	Active participation
	Informal atmosphere
	Broadens perspectives
	We remember what we discuss
	Good for higher-level
	    cognitive, affective objectives
		Learner may be
		    unprepared
		Shy people may not
		    discuss
		May get sidetracked
		More time consuming
		More threatening
		Size of group limited

Projects	More motivating Active participation Good for higher-level cognitive objectives	

Laboratory
    experiments
	Learn by experience
	Hands-on method
	Active participation
	Good for higher-level cognitive
	    objectives
		Requires space, time
		Group size limited

Simulation
    Scenarios
    In-basket
    Role playing
    Critical incidents
	Active participation
	Requires critical thinking
	Develops problem-solving
	    skills
	Connects theory and practice
	More interesting
	Good for higher-level cognitive
	    objectives and affective
	    objectives
		Time consuming
		Group size limited

Demonstration	Realistic
	Appeals to several senses
	Can show a large group
	Good for psychomotor
	    domain
		Requires equipment
		Requires time
		Learner is passive,
		    unless can practice

Source: Holli, B.B. and R.J. Calabrese. *Communication and Education Skills: The Dietitian's Guide.* 2nd ed. Lea & Febiger: Philadelphia; 1991, p. 197.

information is abstract and complex. Learners do not make uniform progress. Research further suggests that men and women may differ in "ways of knowing" and that women may respond better to small-group and experiential-learning activities.

2. Tell learners what they are expected to learn by introducing the key concepts and the most important points in one session.

3. Give a framework for new facts. Outlines, study questions, and study guides help create the framework.

4. Recognize that learners' previous knowledge influences what they learn in a new situation. Learners fit new information into their own familiar framework to give attention to and organize the new material.

5. Relate material to something already meaningful, relevant, or important to the learner. Draw connections between what they already know and what they are learning.

6. Limit the amount of information presented at any one time. New information is absorbed best when presented in small amounts.

7. Broad concepts are understood and remembered and are therefore more meaningful than facts or details.

8. Provide opportunities for active learning. Students learn best by doing, writing, discussing, or taking action. Allow them to summarize, paraphrase, or generalize about the important ideas through group discussion, simulation, case studies, and written assignments.

Instructional Materials

Although the selection of instructional materials follows the development of instructional strategy in the model, it is typically performed during preparation for instruction. The selection of the best materials to use is based on the learning skills desired. If psychomotor skills are expected, specific practice equipment is needed. If attitudinal skills are to be the outcome, visual media is often selected.

In choosing instructional materials, an appropriate first step is to determine if existing materials fill all or part of the needs. Such materials can be examined to determine the appropriate context, sequence, and type of information available. If a video, for instance, fills a specific need toward meeting a session's objective, excerpts of the videotape might be used. Text can be scanned and made into PowerPoint presentations. If appropriate materials are not available, the instructor needs to develop them. If print media is predominantly used, a learner's guide will be helpful. For distance education, much of the instruction is learner-directed and a guide is essential.

Evaluation

Evaluation shows the value or worth of an educational program. The benefits of program evaluation are:[13]

1. Focuses the instructor on the objectives of the instructional program.
2. Provides information for decision making on all aspects of the program.
3. Identifies improvements in the design and delivery of learning events.
4. Increases application of the learning by participants.
5. Provides program accountability and data on the major accomplishments of the program.
6. Identifies ways of improving future programs.

The learning objectives are the basis for evaluation. The evaluation techniques should match the focus of the objectives, such as knowledge acquisition, thinking skills, psychomotor skills, or changes in attitudes, values, or feelings.

Two types of evaluation are used: formative and summative. Formative evaluation is the collection of data during a program. This assists the instructor to improve the instruction while it is underway. Summative evaluation focuses on the results or outcomes of a program.

Use of the Design

The instructional design model presented, with specific steps at each stage, is obviously applied best in the classroom or more formal type of education. However, the concepts presented, such as needs assessment, objectives, instructional strategies and materials, and evaluation should be followed in every presentation, whether formal or informal or with large or small groups. It should be noted that the same process is followed when designing online education, a delivery method that is increasingly used.[14] Elementary through doctoral levels of education and on-the-job training have adapted to using the Inernet as an educational tool. The ADA and many other groups provide continuing education online for members.

EDUCATOR ROLES

"Everything you say or do as well as everything you fail to say will communicate messages. You cannot not influence people."[15] This quote is applicable in whatever role the educator may assume because communicating through verbal interaction and nonverbal cues is characteristic of all roles. Several of these roles are described in the following section.

Mentor

A mentor is a person who teaches by verbal interaction, demonstration of particular activities or skills, and role-modeling. The mentoring relationship is a shared experience between a teacher and a learner. A mentor may be one's peer, an instructor, a trusted advisor, or a younger person—think of the teenager who helps a parent or grandparent become computer literate. The mentor also may be described as a tutor in that both involve one-on-one teaching.

Mentoring has three components: internal trust and commitment from spending time together, patient leadership and time commitment, and emotional maturity.[16] In the workplace, gender or cultural differences can affect the mentoring relationship; hence the need for supervision.

Benefits shown to arise from effective mentoring include the following:[17]

- Increased job skills and job status
- Heightened awareness of organization politics and culture
- Appreciation for and use of networking
- A proactive approach to tasks
- An eagerness to learn
- An attitude of advocacy and willingness to tutor others

A successful statewide mentoring program for dietitians in California resulted in positive feedback from both mentors and mentees. In the program, district training was conducted. The most meaningful outcomes of the training were the following:[18]

- Positive feedback from those mentored
- Help with career change
- Networking and finding mentors through interactions
- The opportunity to provide support to RDs
- Connection of RDs with those who desire to learn new skills

- Opened beneficial new areas of opportunity options
- Informal contacts with students
- Assisted prospective RDs in education plans for RD certification
- Resources available to those interested in the mentoring process

The Nutrition Entrepreneurs Practice Group of the ADA conducts a mentorship program aimed toward matching volunteer mentors with other members who need guidance to make their vision a reality.[19] Bitzer,[20] the mentor program coordinator, points out there are rewards that may be realized by both mentors and those mentored.

Coach

A coach is one who inspires and motivates others. Coaching is sometimes described as the role assumed with individuals who are already achieving at a high level and is simply positive feedback for continued high performance. In actuality, the coaching role is effective only when involvement and trust are created, expectations are clarified, performance is acknowledged, actions are challenged, and achievement is rewarded.[18] The football coach is the classic example of one who performs all these functions in the expectation of having a winning team.

Coaching is similar to "reflective teaching" in that the teacher demonstrates a new procedure or piece of information and the learner listens and learns. The learner performs and the teacher responds with advice, criticism, explanation, description, or further demonstration. The learner "reflects" and compares the new information to his or her previous knowledge and acts accordingly.

Preceptor

The preceptor is one who provides direction and instruction, supervises performance, and evaluates learners in applied practice. The dietitian who oversees a dietetic intern in supervised practice has the title of preceptor. A preceptor must have good interpersonal and time-management skills as well as subject-matter competence as a skilled practitioner. Preceptors are essential in dietetics education and to the future of dietetic practice.

Many benefits are realized by both the preceptors and the students and departments providing experiences for the students. Among the benefits for preceptors observed in one study were:[21] assisting students with application of knowledge and expertise, gaining personal satisfaction, observing students' growth from novice to practitioner, and stimulating ongoing interest in the profession. Students gained valuable knowledge from the example set by experienced professionals and were guided to levels of achievement that allowed them to assume entry-level positions well prepared.

Descriptions of the various roles as perceived by the teacher, preceptor/teacher, preceptor, preceptor/mentor, and mentor are shown in Table 12-3.

Counselor

The role of counselor has two parts: interviewer and counselor. Interviewing involves the gathering of information that is then used to counsel a patient or a client. Counseling is a process of listening, accepting, clarifying, and helping clients form conclusions and develop plans of action. The process is guided by the dietitian toward helping individuals learn about themselves and about methods of coping with their dietary problem.

Motivational interviewing is defined as a way of helping others bring about behavior change, such as curbing addictive behaviors.[22] This technique was used in a study that led to increased fruit and vegetable intake in African Americans.[23] This type of counseling is also described as a "directive, client-centered" style for eliciting behavior change by helping clients explore and resolve ambivalence.

A cognitive interview technique is sometimes used to assist in understanding how audiences or individuals process information. Respondents are led through a survey or message and asked to respond with their thoughts, feelings, or ideas that come to mind. With this information, better messages are formed and valuation tools are targeted.[24]

Patient-centered counseling facilitates change by assessing patient needs and subsequently tailoring the intervention to the patient's stage in the process of change, personal goals, and unique challenges.[25] Four steps are followed: assessment, advising, assisting, and follow-up. In step one, assessment, the dietitian-counselor asks questions to determine present behaviors. Open-ended questions are used for the best results. See Table 12-4 for examples of open-ended questions for each stage of the counseling process.

In step two, personalized advisement based on the assessment is given toward helping a client make changes. Assisting, in step three, involves giving motivational statements and encouragement. Goals and specific skills

Table 12-3. Preceptor Roles

	Teacher	Preceptor/Teacher	Preceptor	Preceptor/Mentor	Mentor
View of intern	View intern as a student[a]		View intern as a prospective coworker[b]		View intern as a colleague[b]
Conceptual focus	Focus on discipline-based learning[b]		Focus on practice-based learning[a]		Focus on personal development[b]
Prior knowledge		Assess intern's prior content knowledge[c]		Assume intern has necessary content knowledge[b]	
Theory/practice	Teach basic subject matter[b]		Demonstrate the incorporation of theory in practice[a]		Identify unwritten workplace policies and practices[b]
Learning experiences	Arrange useful learning experiences to help intern achieve objectives[a]		Suggest useful learning experiences to help intern achieve learning objectives[a]		Encourage intern to determine learning experiences to achieve objectives[c]
Ethical concerns		Discuss potential ethical issues[c]		Identify actual ethical concerns[b]	
Strengths-weaknesses		Identify intern's strengths and weaknesses[a]		Help intern become aware of strengths and weaknesses[a]	

(continues)

Table 12-3. Preceptor Roles (*continued*)

	Teacher	Preceptor/Teacher	Preceptor	Preceptor/Mentor	Mentor
Progress evaluation	Provide intern with an evaluation of academic progress[c]			Provide intern with an evaluation of professional progress[a]	
Intern self-evaluation			Identify usefulness of self-evaluation[c]		Strongly encourage intern to participate in self-evaluation[c]
Role model	View yourself as an academic role model[a]		View yourself as a professional role model[a]		View yourself as a personal role model[a]
Duration of relationship		Recognize relationship with intern is limited[a]			View the relationship with the intern as indefinite[b]

Columns represent the categorical descriptions for each role. Rows represent the functions/elements that relate to the supervised practice experience. [a]Practices preceptors indicated they "frequently" execute and do not want to change. [b]Practices preceptors executed in varying degrees from frequently or occasionally to seldom/never, but do not want to change. [c]Practice preceptors believed they should do more often.

Source: Wilson, M.A. "Dietetic Preceptors Perceive Their Role to Include a Variety of Elements." *J Am Diet Assoc* 102, no. 7(2002): 969.

Table 12-4. A Model for Open-Ended Questioning

Questions for Assessing Stage of Change and Motivation

How do you feel about your current diet?

What problems have you had because of your diet?

What would you like to change about your diet now?

Why would you like to change your diet now?

What concerns do you have about changing your diet now?

What reasons might you have to want to maintain your current diet?

What would motivate you to maintain your current diet?

Questions for Assessing Past Experiences with Dietary Change

What changes have you made to your diet? How long did you maintain the changes? If so, for how long? If not, how long did you maintain the change?

How did you make changes in your diet? What helped?

What difficulties did you encounter? How did you handle them?

Questions about Anticipated Challenges or Barriers to Change

What could get in your way of attaining your goal?

What situations will make it hardest for you to achieve your goal?

What other situations might make it difficult for you to maintain your change?

Questions about Strategies to Cope with Challenges or Barriers to Change

What could you do when you face this challenge?

What else could you do in the face of this challenge or barrier?

Who could help you cope with this challenge? How?

What has been helpful in the past to deal with this barrier?

Questions for Goal Setting

What are you willing to change in your diet now?

When? How often will you do this?

Where will you do it?

What will you have to do in advance to ensure that you are able to make and maintain this change?

How confident are you of your ability to make and maintain this change?

Questions for Follow-Up

How did you do with your plan?

What helped you stay on target?

What difficulties did you encounter?

Questions for Assessing Lapse and Relapse

What made it difficult for you to stay with your plan?

How did you feel after that?

What else could you have done to stay on track?

What would you like to do now?

Source: Rosal, M.C., C.B. Ebbeling, I. Lofgren, J.K. Ockene, I.S. Ockene, and J.R. Hebert. "Facilitating Dietary Change: The Patient-Centered Counseling Model." *J Am Diet Assoc* 101, no. 3(2001): 333.

such as self-monitoring and other problem solving will also be discussed. In the final step, follow-up toward maintaining dietary changes will be presented. In this stage, the attainment of the earlier goals will be discussed and further help offered. Again, open-ended questions are used.

Communicator

Effective communication is of utmost importance in all areas of dietetics, and almost any job description will include the need to communicate at all levels in an organization as well as with individuals. Professionals who develop verbal and written skills, along with listening skills, establish stronger relationships with clients, patients, and staff.

There are, at a minimum, seven components of the communication process. They are as follows:

1. The source is the starting point for information exchange.
2. The message is the idea or information transmitted verbally or nonverbally.
3. The channel is the pathway for messages between the sender and the receiver.
4. The receiver takes in the message, assigns meaning, interprets, and responds to the message.
5. Feedback refers to the response from the receiver to the sender.

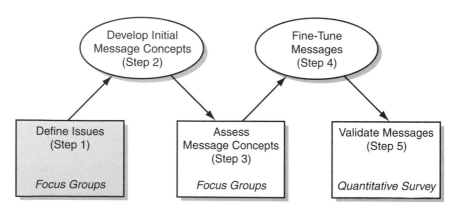

FIGURE 12-1. The Consumer Message Development Model.

Source: Borra, S., L. Kelly, M. Tuttle, and K. Neville. "Developing Actionable Dietary Guidance Messages: Dietary Fat as a Case Study." *J Am Diet Assoc* 101, no. 6(2001): 679.

6. The environment is the context in which the message occurs, such as physical surrounding, cultural, historic, or attitudinal factors.
7. Noise is any aural, visual, or internal factor that can distract from the meaning of the message.

The communication methods that ensure messages are received need to be carefully selected. Professionals who provide nutrition information to the public will choose methods such as television, Internet, or printed materials.

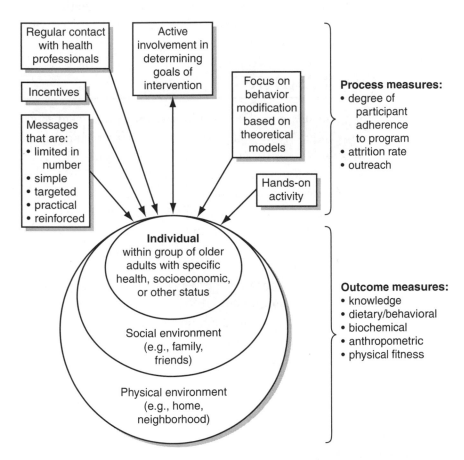

FIGURE 12-2. A Framework for Designing a Nutrition Education Intervention for Older Adults.

Source: Sayhoun, N.R., C.A. Pratt, and A. Anderson. "Evaluation of Nutrition Education Interventions for Older Adults: A Proposed Framework." *J Am Diet Assoc* 104, no. 1(2004): 66.

The development of actionable dietary guidance messages through use of focus groups and surveys of consumers is described by Borra.[26] In the consumer message development model (Figure 12-1), the issues are defined, the message developed and assessed, then fine-tuned, and validated.

In another study to determine the best means of communicating nutrition education for elderly adults, several factors were found to be successful.[27] They included limiting educational messages to one or two; reinforcing and personalizing messages; providing purposeful activities and incentives; providing access to health professionals; and using appropriate theories of behavior change. A model was developed incorporating these elements. Figure 12-2 demonstrates application of this model to designing a nutrition education intervention for older adults.

TYPES OF LEARNING

Education through the use of methods that involve the learner in an active, participatory way can lead to very effective outcomes. Internships are examples of one type: service learning. Problem-based learning (PBL) is the method by which a student discovers new knowledge through individual effort. Project-based learning, similar to problem-based, is the method in which learner involvement is guided by an instructor. These three types of learning are described in the following sections.

Service Learning

Service learning is a type of educational experience that combines explicit academic learning with community service.[28] In many professions, the idea of combining classroom study and community learning experiences is thought to enhance and retain learning. In dietetics, the internship is an example of service learning in that it combines practice with instruction. Another example is the college class that places students in a community site such as a school or elderly nutrition program for experiences that are a part of the course requirement. Seeing and experiencing nutrition applied in specific community programs makes subject matter come alive and leads to a better understanding of the value and need of community service.

Problem-Based Learning

A method used successfully in medical and business schools, problem-based learning calls students to work through problems to find answers to real-life situations. PBL provides a context for students to learn critical thinking and problem-solving skills and to acquire knowledge of the essential concepts of a course of study.[29] In this method, students are presented a problem and organized into groups to discuss the problem. Students pose questions and rank the learning issues generated in the session. Students and the instructor discuss the resources needed to research the learning issues. Students then summarize their knowledge and connect the new concepts to older ones and define new learning issues as they progress through the problem. The benefit is that students recognize that learning is an ongoing process with new learning issues to be explored.

The role of the instructor in PBL is to guide, probe, and support students' initiatives. When faculty incorporate PBL wholly or in part into classes, they empower students to take a responsible role in their learning. As a result, faculty must be ready to yield some authority to their students.

Project-Based learning

Similar to PBL, project-based learning is a form of instruction that places emphasis on the students' involvement in working through job-related situations. It is described as long-term, problem-focused, meaningful units of instruction that integrate concepts from a number of disciplines. An example might be the design of a kitchen layout using work flow, equipment, and production schedules. Both teachers and students receive support in fulfilling their roles, the teacher as facilitator and "shepherd" of projects, and the students by participating in a whole project. A project-based learning support system has been described that supports learning through a computer-mediated interface using learner-centered software.[30] This type of learning is useful in simulations or when students share a concentrated experience, as in an internship. New tools and structures are often needed to support the effectiveness of this type of learning, but it provides good results amid complex and challenging projects.

ADULTS AS LEARNERS

Conducting learning sessions for adults is different than for teaching younger people. Dietitians need to be aware of the differences in order to adapt their teaching for the best learning outcomes. Holli and Calabrese[31] describe five assumptions about adult learners as follows:

1. Adults are independent and self-directed by their own preference.
2. Adults have backgrounds of experience that can be used as a resource for learning.
3. The adult's readiness to learn is based on desire to learn social roles and to solve problems.
4. Adult learning is oriented toward performing tasks and solving problems because adults typically have an immediate need for the information.
5. Adults are motivated by internal cues such as recognition, self-esteem, or personal satisfaction. They usually learn best when they are active participants in planning and implementing the learning experiences in which they will be involved.

TEACHING GROUPS AND TEAMS

Groups of people act in ways that are different than when they are in a one-on-one learning situation. Group dynamics is a term often applied to this behavior because it describes how members relate to each other, how they communicate among themselves, and how they work as a group.[32] The teacher or leader of the group needs to understand how these dynamics can affect the learning process and the ways the educational message needs to be delivered.

Some of the skills needed for working with and teaching groups include the following:

1. Groups function best when all members participate and contribute ideas. The instructor can help this happen by encouraging and coaching.
2. Sharing information within the group helps to ensure that all have the same knowledge. Asking questions and initiating open discussion are ways of sharing.
3. All members of the group must understand the subject or the task. This may mean that the instructor or other group members add examples or explanations to make the information clear to all. This also may be accomplished by showing how the ideas and activities of two or more of the group are related and coordinated.

4. The instructor or leader needs to orient the group to the purpose and expected outcomes of the learning situation. Goals are clarified and direction provided that leads the discussion.
5. When verbal or other support is given for ideas and participation, the group is more likely to accept and learn. Encouraging discussion rather than debate usually leads to suggestions for new solutions and helps avoid members of the group "taking sides."
6. Recognizing that conflict and tension can arise in groups can help members and the leader be prepared to inject humor or take other means to reduce tension. A time-out or a temporary change of subject may accomplish this.
7. Another technique, gatekeeping, refers to being alert to signals that members of the group send about wanting to speak or otherwise participate. All members of the group should have an equal opportunity to be heard; at the same time, some may need to be encouraged to express themselves if they have not been active participants.

While teams are focused as a work group, many of the same characteristics as evidenced in groups will also appear. Teams may be formed in order to accomplish more through the combined efforts and expertise of individual members. Participation in teams, however, requires that members understand their role and the expectations for the group.

When teams are first formed, members may be uncertain of their role and will depend on a leader to guide them into a team role. There may be conflict as team members clarify the team's goals. The leader then needs to redirect the energies of the team by encouraging open communication. As relationships become cohesive, the team functions as a unit and develops patterns of communication and behavior. The leader facilitates decision making and problem solving. The team members find ways of handling conflict, and methods therefore develop that become standards for evaluating team performance. Finally, the team prepares for a change: regrouping, a change in leader, or a change in the goals for which the group was formed.

SUMMARY

The role of educator is one of the most important of those performed by the dietitian and dietetic technician. To be an effective educational leader, the professional must have a working knowledge of the education process by assessing learners' foundational knowledge, setting learning goals, planning learning content and delivery methods, and evaluating the outcomes of the learning.

The dietitian may function in a number of educator roles, including mentor, coach, preceptor, or counselor. The effective teacher in any of these roles is skilled in communications and has the qualities of a leader in understanding individuals and groups and fostering productive working relationships.

DEFINITIONS

Assessment. The process of evaluating actions or conditions on which to base further activity.

Cognitive Skills. The application of intellectual capabilities to accomplish objectives.

Domain of Learning. A group or category of ideas, learning strategies, or classification system.

Education. The systematic instruction and training designed to impart knowledge and develop a skill.

Instruction. The activity by which knowledge or teaching is imparted.

Psychomotor Skills. The ability to perform physical tasks based on knowing or thinking.

Supervision. The process of directing the work, workers, or the operation of an organization.

Training. Actions by which persons are brought to a desired standard of efficiency or behavior by instruction and practice.

REFERENCES

1. Puckett, R.P. "Education and the Dietetics Profession." *J Am Diet Assoc* 97, no. 3(1997): 252–253.
2. Kane, M.T., A.S. Cohen, E.R. Smith, C. Lewis, and C. Reidy. "1995 Commission on Dietetic Registration Dietetics Practice Audit." *J Am Diet Assoc* 96(1996): 1292–1301.
3. Roach, R.R., J.W. Pichert, B.A. Stetson, R.A. Lorenz, E.J. Boswell, and D.G. Schlundt. "Improving Dietitian's Teaching Skills." *J Am Diet Assoc* 92, no. 12(1992): 1466–1473.

4. Holli, B.B. and R.J. Calabrese. *Communication and Education Skills: The Dietitian's Guide.* 2nd ed. Lea & Febiger: Philadelphia; 1991, pp. 174–176.
5. Gagne, R.M. *Instructional Technology: Foundations.* Lawrence Erlbaum Associates: Hillsdale, NJ; 1987, p. 25.
6. Mager, R.F. *Preparing Instructional Objectives.* 2nd ed. David S. Lake Publisher: Belmont, CA; 1984, p. 183.
7. Bloom, B.S., M. Engehard, E. Furet, W. Hill, and D. Krathwohl. *Taxonomy of Educational Objectives. Handbook 1: Cognitive Domain.* David McKay: New York; 1956, pp. 20–21.
8. See Note 7.
9. Krathwohl, D., B.S. Bloom, and B. Masia. *Taxonomy of Educational Objectives. Handbook II: Affective Domain.* David McKay: New York; 1964.
10. Simpson, E. "The Classification of Educational Objectives in the Psychomotor Domain." *Illinois Teacher of Home Economics* 10(1966): 110.
11. See Note 5.
12. Davis, B.G. *Tools for Teaching.* Jossey-Bass: San Francisco; 1993, p. 45.
13. Caffarelli, R.S. *Planning Programs for Adult Learners.* Jossey-Bass: San Francisco; 1994, p. 120.
14. Sandon, L. "A System for Designing Effective Online Education." *J Am Diet Assoc* 107, no. 8(2007): 1305–1306.
15. Hendricks, W., ed. *Coaching, Mentoring and Managing.* Career Press: Franklin Lakes, NJ; 1996.
16. Kaye, B. and B. Jackson. "Reframing Mentoring." *Training and Development* 50(1996): 44–47.
17. See Note 15.
18. Schatz, P.E., T.J. Bush-Zurn, C. Aresa, and K.C. Freeman. "California's Professional Mentoring Program: How to Develop a Statewide Mentoring Program." *J Am Diet Assoc* 103, no. 1(2003): 73–76.
19. Bitzer, R. "Mentor Program." Nutrition Entrepreneurs Practice Group. *Ventures* XXV, no. 4(2009): 11.
20. Bitzer, R. "Mentor Program." Nutrition Entrepreneurs Practice Group. *Ventures* XXV, no. 5(2009): 8.
21. Marincic, P.Z. and E.E. Francfort. "Supervised Program Preceptors' Perceptions of Rewards, Benefits, Support, and Commitment to the Preceptor Role." *J Am Diet Assoc* 102, no. 4(2002): 543–545.
22. Thorpe, M. "Motivational Interviewing and Dietary Behavior Change." *J Am Diet Assoc* 103, no. 2(2003): 150–151.
23. Resicow, K., A. Jackson, T. Wang, F. McCarty, W.W. Dudley, and T. Baranowski. "A Motivational Interviewing Intervention to Increase Fruit and Vegetable Intake Through Black Churches: Results of the Eat for Life Trial." *Am J Pub Health* 91(2001): 1686–1693.
24. Carbone, E.T., M.K. Campbell, and L. Honess-Morreal. "Use of Cognitive Interview Techniques in the Development of Nutrition Surveys and Interactive

Messages for Low-Income Populations." *J Am Diet Assoc* 102, no. 5(2002): 690–696.

25. Rosal, M.C., C.B. Ebbeling, I. Lofgren, J.K. Ockene, I.S. Ockene, and J.R. Hebert. "Facilitating Dietary Change: The Patient-Centered Counseling Model." *J Am Diet Assoc* 101, no. 3(2001): 332–341.

26. Borra, S., L. Kelly, M. Tuttle, and K. Neville. "Developing Actionable Dietary Guidance Messages: Dietary Fat as a Case Study." *J Am Diet Assoc* 101, no. 6(2001): 678–684.

27. Sayhoun, N.R., C.A. Pratt, and A. Anderson. "Evaluation of Nutrition Education Interventions for Older Adults: A Proposed Framework." *J Am Diet Assoc* 104, no. 1(2004): 58–69.

28. Kim, Y. and A. Canfield. "How to Develop a Service Learning Program in Dietetics Education." *J Am Diet Assoc* 102, no. 2(2002): 174–176.

29. Dietetic Educators of Practitioners Practice Group. "Problem-Based Learning: Preparing Students to Succeed in the 21st Century." *DEP Line* 17, no. 3(1998): 1–5.

30. Laffey, J., T. Tupper, D. Musser, and J. Wedman. "A Computer-Mediated Support for Project-Based Learning." *Technology Research and Development* 46, no. 1(1998): 73–86.

31. See Note 4.

32. See Note 4.

CHAPTER 13

Research in Dietetics

"As a profession, the one thing we can predict is that the greatest changes in our practice will be the change in knowledge and how we integrate new science into our daily practice."[1]

OUTLINE

- Introduction
- Importance of Research in Dietetics
- ADA Research Philosophy
- ADA Research Priorities
  - ADA Research Committee
  - Research Dietetic Practice Group
- Research Applications
- Career Opportunities in Research
  - Academic Health Centers
  - Food and Industry Companies
  - Government
  - Community and Public Health
  - Nutrition Research Centers
- Research Activities and Funding
- Summary

INTRODUCTION

Much of the research in nutrition and dietetics is conducted by students and faculty members at colleges and universities. Some of these researchers are Registered Dietitians; others are food, nutrition, or allied scientists. Most faculty members both teach and conduct research as part of their faculty responsibilities. They may conduct laboratory research, such as metabolic studies in human nutrient requirements or in food science to determine utilization of specific food components. Other studies may be conducted in controlled working environments as, for example, in food service management productivity studies. Other kinds of research may deal with applied studies in nutrition education and data collection through surveys.

With the ADA's increasing emphasis on research and research funding, many dietitians are incorporating research studies into their practice. In part, there is a sense that more applied research is needed as higher-level academic research does not always meet the needs of everyday practice. To this end, a member-network has been formed called the Dietetics Practice-Based Research Network (DPBRN).[2] The network is open to all who are interested in addressing questions encountered in practice, and to continually improve the delivery of food and nutrition services.

The DPBRN brings practitioners and researchers together to identify research that is needed in practice settings, to design significant research, to obtain funding, and to carry the research into real-life practice. The focus of the research conducted by members is on studies that can be immediately incorporated into practice. Professionals who lack the time, money, or expertise to conduct research find this group activity presents an opportunity to benefit from research by answering questions and keeping abreast of new information.

IMPORTANCE OF RESEARCH IN DIETETICS

"Well-designed and well-conducted research is critical for our profession, as it produces the scientific evidence upon which dietetics practice is based."[3] Any profession needs to continually reshape itself to meet ever-changing needs in society, and therefore research is essential for advancement in the profession. Not only do dietitians need to engage in research to uncover new knowledge and define new modes of therapy, but they also need to take a scholarly approach to everyday practice. As Parks[4] and others have pointed out:

> To ensure that our clients receive only the very best dietetics care, we must develop aptitudes and attitudes for scholarship; question underlying assumptions to our knowledge base and to our practice; be curious about how science can be used to make us better practitioners and have the courage to challenge the very essence of our current knowledge.

Employers of dietitians or those using dietetic services want to be assured that the services they are using are supported by research. Research is the basis for education because it drives the core knowledge and competencies and is used in setting public policy. The ability to conduct and use research further allows professionals to be recognized by the public as a valued and credible source of scientific nutrition information.

ADA RESEARCH PHILOSOPHY

The research philosophy of the profession is the following:

> The ADA believes that research is the foundation of the profession, providing the basis for practice, education, and policy. Dietetics is the integration and application of principles derived from the sciences of nutrition, biochemistry, physiology, food management, and behavioral and social sciences to achieve and maintain people's health; therefore dietetics research is a dynamic collaborative and assimilative endeavor. This research is broad in scope, ranging from basic to applied practice research.[5]

ADA RESEARCH PRIORITIES

ADA Research Committee

The research committee, reporting to the Board of Directors and the House of Delegates, sets the research agenda for the Association. In this capacity, the committee develops, maintains, and evaluates the research agenda for the Association.[6] The ADA's statement of purpose emphasizes research: "ADA is committed to improving the nation's health and advancing the profession of dietetics through research, education, and advocacy." Two specific strategies to help reach these goals are the following:

1. Equip members to use research in their work.
2. Provide research and resources that can be translated into evidence-based practice.

The research agenda of the ADA identifies research priorities in the areas of dietetics, nutrition, behavioral and social science, management, basic science, and food science. Descriptions of each of these research areas follow:

Behavioral and social science research: Research that examines effective nutrition and lifestyle education, communication, and behavior change strategies for prevention and treatment of obesity and chronic or acute disease.

Food science research: Research to examine ways to improve, evaluate, and provide access to a safe, culturally appropriate, sustainable food and water supply to protect the health of the public.

Basic physiology and nutrition research: Research that explores the interactions among diet, genetics, metabolomics, proteomics, and transcriptomics.

Nutrition care process: Research that examines the components of the nutrition care process, including methods for nutrition assessment, validity of nutrition diagnosis, effect of nutrition interventions, and identification of appropriate health outcome measures for individuals and populations.

Delivery of dietetic services: Research to develop effective methods for delivery of dietetic services and payment for the services.

Dietetics and retention: Research that examines the best methods for attracting, educating, and retaining competent ADA members and credentialed Registered Dietitians and Dietetic Technicians, Registered.

The Research Committee of the ADA identifies the priority research areas as core research and dietetics-specific research.[7] The core priorities for the Association are:

1. Nutrition and lifestyle-change intervention to prevent or treat obesity and chronic diseases
2. Safe, secure, and sustainable food supply
3. Nutrients and systems biology (nutrigenetics and nutrigenomics)

The dietetics-specific research priorities are:

1. Nutrition care process and health outcome measures
2. Delivery and reimbursement of dietetic services
3. Dietetics education and retention

Funding for approved projects comes from the ADA Foundation and other ADA-affiliated groups, from governmental agencies, and from the food and nutrition industry.

The research committee is developing a research toolkit to aid persons new to research. The toolkit will provide a lesson or tutorial, practice suggestions, and resources for conducting research.[8]

Research Dietetic Practice Group

The Research Dietetic Practice Group has over 650 members from a variety of work settings, including clinical research centers, nonprofit groups, governmental agencies, universities, and many practice areas. Membership is open to all ADA members who conduct research or are interested in research. Members collaborate on Association projects, such as the Evidence Analysis Library, to bring together research from many sources, and in the preparation of Position Papers. Members also form liaisons with the ADA Research Committee and the DPBRN. The practice group also provides a member network; conducts continuing professional education events; provides a packet of information for new members; and produces a Web site and *The Venture*, a periodic publication for members. Research awards are given to recognize the research and publications generated by members.

RESEARCH APPLICATIONS

Evidence-based practice is the integration of the best available evidence from reviewed research with professional expertise and client values to make food and nutrition practice decisions.[9] Every area of practice in dietetics involves making decisions about best procedures to follow and, given that new information continually leads to a need to make necessary changes or to update practice, evidence analysis provides this information. The evidence analysis process involves the following steps:

1. Formulate one or more questions to be researched.
2. Conduct a literature review for each question.

3. Critically appraise each report found in the literature as to the quality of the research and the findings.
4. Summarize the evidence.
5. Develop conclusions and assign a grade based on the strength of the evidence.
6. Put into practice.

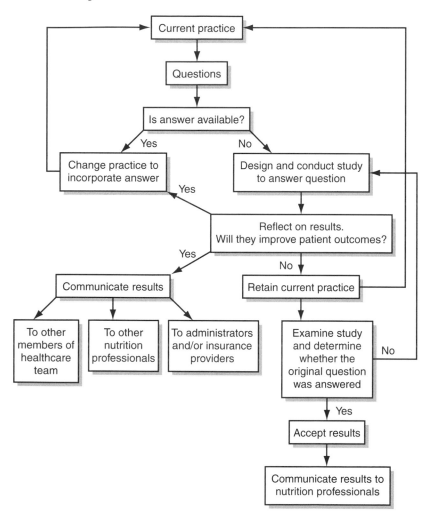

FIGURE 13-1. Detailed Progression of How Research and Clinical Practice Are Integrated.

Source: Eck, L.H., D.O. Slawson, R. Williams, K. Smith, K. Harmon-Clayton, and D. Oliver. "A Model for Making Outcomes Research Standard Practice in Clinical Dietetics." *J Am Diet Assoc* 98, no. 4(1998): 455.

The Evidence Analysis Library at the ADA headquarters office is maintained for the benefit of members of the Association and others needing the information. The best and most relevant nutrition information is reviewed and is available in an accessible, online, user-friendly library.[10] Because of the research data held, governmental and other groups also use the information and the process in making policy decisions. One example group is the Food and Drug Administration who use the process to make decisions about the use of health claims on food labels.

Outcomes research is increasingly important in the linkage of practice and research in order to make advancements in all areas of dietetics. Surveys show that while dietitians consider research important and are interested in it, many experience obstacles to performing outcomes research because of lack of research knowledge and skills, along with limited time and funding.[11,12] Eck and colleagues[13] proposed a model for incorporating outcomes research in clinical dietetics (Figure 13-1). Hayes and Peterson[14] advocate a training curriculum to enhance professionals' understanding of research.

CAREER OPPORTUNITIES IN RESEARCH

Academic Health Centers

Many university-affiliated hospitals have centers dedicated to types of clinical research. Others have long-term multidisciplinary research projects that include a nutrition component. Some dietitians work at a general clinical research center (GCRC), usually associated with an academic medical center and federally funded. There are about 80 GCRCs funded by the National Institutes of Health (NIH) located at universities such as Ohio State, Emory, Stanford, Rockefeller, and University of Iowa.

Research dietitians may oversee the metabolic kitchens associated with the GCRCs, analyze nutrient intakes, conduct calorimetry studies, assist in development of nutrition-related protocols, and participate in rounds and seminars.

Some GCRC dietitians manage their own research programs, direct clinical nutrition research, and collaborate with the medical school faculty in research in areas such as diabetes, cancer, and others. Some large national studies provide numerous opportunities for dietitians to become involved as nutrition counselors, data managers, or project directors.

The need for dietitians involved in clinical research continues. The best dietetics practice must be based on scientific principles and sound theory. However, more evidence is needed to support the value of many approaches to clinical dietetics. Additional knowledge is needed in areas of nutritional status of individuals and populations at risk for disease, identification of nutrient requirements associated with disease conditions, and nutrition interventions as therapy for disease conditions. With the crises in healthcare delivery, the outcomes of nutrition intervention are an important area of investigation.

Food and Industry Companies

Many food companies employ dietitians. Roles vary but include research related to product or recipe development. Roles can also focus on translation of research into meaningful information for the public or development of nutrition education for children, adults, and professionals.

Companies that manufacture infant formulas and medical nutritional products often employ dietitians to conduct research or to monitor clinical investigations in hospitals, nursing homes, and home care settings. Roles might include work related to:

- Nutritional needs of infants, children, and the elderly
- Acceptability of flavors and textures of products designed for oral use
- Coordination of studies to determine the effectiveness of new products
- Initiation of outcomes research to explore the cost-effectiveness of medical nutrition therapy

Government

There are many opportunities for research dietitians in government-sponsored centers and laboratories. These include positions such as:

- Nutrition scientist at the Department of Agriculture laboratories studying nutrient requirements, vitamins and minerals, and the like
- Researcher at the U.S. Army Natick Research, Development, and Engineering Center in Massachusetts involved in studies related to food behaviors and the acceptance and consumption of military rations
- Nutrition epidemiologist at the Centers for Disease Control in Atlanta exploring patterns of nutrition-related diseases throughout the country
- Extension specialist at a land-grant university exploring ways to maximize food production, quality, and safety

- Life science specialist at the Congressional Research Service in the Library of Congress, answering questions and conducting research for members of Congress and staff on food safety and nutrition issues
- Nutrition researcher at the National Aeronautical and Space Administration in Houston studying nutrition needs of space explorers

Community and Public Health

Since the leading causes of death in the United States continue to be nutrition-related chronic dieases, more efforts and opportunities are arising in community- and population-based nutrition research. As consumers become more aware of disease consequences of their food choices and eating behaviors, they demand more evidence of science-based causes and effects. Many dietitians who previously worked only in service program areas in community and public health are seizing the opportunity for research activities that document the value of nutrition and the dietitians' role in interventions.

Schools are involved in research especially suited for nutrition, healthy behaviors, and weight maintenance by providing researchers access to students that they can follow over time. Dietitians will be needed in greater numbers for these research and education programs to be successful.

Many land-grant universities are conducting nutrition research in developing countries around the world. This research involves food and agriculture production, economic development, and nutritional assessment and intervention in various populations. As more and more globalization occurs, these ventures will increase, thus providing ever greater opportunities for dietitians in research.

Nutrition Research Centers

The Agricultural Research Service of the U.S. Department of Agriculture funds six human nutrition research centers. These include the Children's Nutrition Research Center at Baylor College of Medicine in Houston and the Arkansas Children's Nutrition Center at Arkansas Children's Hospital at the University of Arkansas for Medical Sciences. The Center at Boston specializes in nutrition research for the aging population and is associated with Tufts University. Located on the campus of the University of California at Davis, the Western Human Nutrition Research Center concentrates on nutrition intervention strategies. The Center at Beltsville, Maryland, conducts basic and applied research on nutrient composition, national dietary surveys, nutrient requirement, function of physiochemicals, and similar studies. The sixth center, located in Grand Forks, North Dakota, is associated with the University of North Dakota and has research interest in mineral requirements and utilization as well as community-based research with Native Americans.

RESEARCH ACTIVITIES AND FUNDING

For information about types of research and research methodology, an excellent source is *Research: Successful Approaches*.[15] The *Journal of the American Dietetic Association* publishes articles about types of research,[16] publishing research,[17,18] funding, and scientific integrity.[19] A series of articles on publishing nutrition research and types of nutrition research provides almost a complete primer on the elements of research and preparing research results for publication.[20–22]

SUMMARY

Researchers may be based in specialized clinical research centers, government agencies, industry, universities, or the workplace. Roles vary according to the employing institution's mission and purpose. Key areas of investigation relate to nutrient requirements, food and specialized nutritional products, nutrient utilization, and outcomes of medical nutrition therapy. Opportunities for participating in outcomes research in order to enhance practice exist through collaborative research that utilizes the expertise of dietitians in many practice settings. All dietitians can benefit from research findings applied to practice through the Evidence Analysis Library of the ADA.

DEFINITIONS

Academic Health Center. Hospital, medical center, or clinic affiliated with a medical school or medical residency program.
Medical Nutrition Education. Basic and applied nutrition for medical students or residents. This often requires integration of concepts related to food science, nutrition, biochemistry, physiology, pathophysiology, health promotion, and human behavior.

Evidence-Based Research. The compilation of research studies that, together, allow for a decision regarding application to practice.

Outcomes Research. Studies that focus on results and application of the results of research.

Research. Systematic investigation leading to new knowledge or new applications of known information. To conduct research, a question is formulated, a literature search conducted, experimental activities applied, and results recorded.

REFERENCES

1. Park, S., R. Schiller, and J.L. Bryk. "President's Page: Investment in Our Future—The Role of Science and Scholarship in Developing Knowledge for Dietetics Practice." *J Am Diet Assoc* 94, no. 10(1994): 1159–1161.
2. Trostler, N., E.F, Meyer, and L.G. Snetselaar. "Description of Practice Characteristics and Professional Activities of Dietetics Practice-Based Research Network Members." *J Am Diet Assoc* 108, no. 6(2008): 1060–1067.
3. Monsen, E.L. and L. Van Horn. "Research: The Foundation of Practice." *J Am Diet Assoc* 103, no. 7(1994): 1159–1161.
4. See Note 1.
5. ADA. "Priorities for Research: Agenda to Support the Future of Dietetics." 2007. www.eatright.org/ada/files/ADA_Priority_for_Research.2007.pdf (Accessed December 3, 2009).
6. Krummel, D. "Research at the Association Level." In *The Digest.* Publication of Research Dietetic Practice Group. Fall 2008.
7. See Note 5.
8. See Note 6.
9. Vaughn, L.A. and C.J.K. Manning. "Meeting the Challenges of Dietetics Practice with Evidence-Based Decisions." *J Am Diet Assoc* 104, no. 2(2004): 282–284.
10. ADA. "Evidence Based Library." www.eatright.org (Accessed April 10, 2009).
11. McCaffree, J. "Overcoming Obstacles to Outcomes Research." *J Am Diet Assoc* 102, no. 1(2002): 71.
12. Hayes, J.E. and C.A. Peterson. "Use of an Outcomes Research Collaborative Training Curriculum to Enhance Entry-Level Dietitians and Established Professionals' Self-Reported Understanding of Research." *J Am Diet Assoc* 103, no. 1(2003): 77–81.
13. Eck, L.H., D.O. Slawson, R. Williams, K. Smith, K. Harmon-Clayton, and D. Oliver. "A Model for Making Outcomes Research Standards Practice in Clinical Dietetics." *J Am Diet Assoc* 98, no. 4(1998): 451–457.
14. See Note 12.
15. Monsen, E.R. and L. Van Horn. *Research: Successful Approaches.* 3rd ed. American Dietetic Association: Chicago, IL; 2007.

16. Harris, J.E., G.P.M. Gleason, P.M. Sheean, C. Boushey, J.A. Beto, and B. Bruemmer. "An Introduction to Qualitative Research for Food and Nutrition Professionals." *J Am Diet Assoc* 109, no. 1(2009): 80–90.

17. Boushey, C., J. Harris, B. Bruemmer, S.L. Archer, and L. Van Horn. "Publishing Nutrition Research: A Review of Study Design, Statistical Analyses, and Other Key Elements of Manuscript Preparation, Part 1." *J Am Diet Assoc* 106, no. 1(2006): 89–96.

18. Harris, J.E., C. Boushey, B. Bruemmer, and S.A. Archer. "Publishing Nutrition Research: A Review of Nonparametric Methods, Part 3." *J Am Diet Assoc* 108, no. 9(2008): 1488–1496.

19. The International Life Sciences Institute (ILSE) North America Conflict of Interest/Scientific Integrity Guiding Principles Working Group. "Funding Food Science and Nutrition Research: Financial Conflicts and Scientific Integrity." *J Am Diet Assoc* 109, no. 5(2009): 929–936.

20. See Note 18.

21. See Note 17.

22. Boushey, C., J. Harris, B. Bruemmer, and S.L. Archer. "Publishing Nutrition Research: A Review of Sampling, Sample Size, Statistical Analyses, and Other Key Elements of Manuscript Preparation. Part 2. " *J Am Diet Assoc* 108, no. 5(2008): 679–688.

Part V

The Future

CHAPTER 14

The Future in Dietetics

"The dogma of the quiet past are inadequate for the stormy present and future. As our circumstances are new, we must think anew, and act anew."[1]
Abraham Lincoln

OUTLINE

- Introduction
- Changing Demographics
- Trends and Issues
  - Ethnic Diversity
  - Age Diversity
  - Aging Population
  - Health and Wellness
  - Communications
  - Environmental Issues
  - Nutrigenomics and Nanotechnology
- Changing Roles in the Healthcare System
- Implications and Challenges for the Profession
- Competition and Collaboration with Other Professions
- Competencies of the Future Dietetics Professional
- Future Roles for the Profession
  - Opportunities in Health Care
  - Food
  - Information Technology and Management
  - Research
  - Public Service
  - Planning for the Future
- Summary

INTRODUCTION

As the dietetics profession progresses into the 21st century, the challenges faced earlier are true today. The new millennium brings a hypercompetitive healthcare environment greatly altered by new information technologies, business practices, managed care and integrated healthcare systems, and changing consumer demands. Clearly, the dietetic profession, like all health professions, is in a time of unprecedented volatility and change.

A growing number of driving forces will dramatically reshape the profession. Among the most significant trends are changing demographics, growing globalization, increasing consumer expectations, a merging knowledge economy, technological revolution, and a restructured workforce. To be competitive in a rapidly changing environment will require a proactive understanding of changing healthcare markets, development of new global competencies and capabilities, and a shift from tangible assets to an appreciation of the value of knowledge and technology. Professions aspiring to make a difference in the lives of individuals will be playing a different game—competing for the future.

CHANGING DEMOGRAPHICS

Demographic factors define healthcare markets from three perspectives: composition, accessibility, and mobility. Two significant demographic influences on healthcare delivery are the aging population and ethnic diversity. The coming years will be characterized by a rapidly increasing number of elderly who will dramatically shift the focus of health services from acute to chronic care, which will likely strain the whole healthcare system.

Accessibility of health care will continue to be a problem unless governmental changes are made. At present, due to high healthcare costs, a large percentage of the U.S. population continues to be without adequate health care. Growing poverty among the nation's rural population, ethnic groups, and at-risk elderly is not likely to improve and will place additional demands on the healthcare system. This gap between the "haves" and "have nots" will likely continue to broaden.

Another significant characteristic of the U.S. healthcare market is mobility. Women continue to move into the workforce and are no longer available to care for aging parents. Extended family members have relocated to distances too far away to provide support to family members with acute and chronic diseases. Even those individuals within a geographic region are mobile. Of the 37 million American professionals employed outside the home, 75 percent are away from their offices at least 1 day a week. These individuals will buy time and convenience, along with health products and services, and will demand "on-the-go" services.

TRENDS AND ISSUES

Ethnic Diversity

Among the diverse ethnic groups in the United States, Latinos are the fastest growing minority group. From 15 percent of the U.S. population in 2009, this population is expected to increase to about 25 percent of the population by 2050.[2] Compared with whites, Latinos experience significantly higher rates of poverty, food insecurity, depression, lack of leisure time and related physical activity, obesity, and diabetes.[3] A study of acculturation and diet among Latinos, principally in California, concluded that the less acculturated may need more stress on dietary choices and food preparation practices while the more acculturated may benefit from messages that stress moderation of fast food, sugar-sweetened beverages, and other away-from-home foods.[4]

Ethnic foods, cultural practices, and language all present challenges for health professionals working with persons with different ethnic backgrounds. Knowledge about nutritional values of ethnic foods, understanding of cultural views on health and nutrition in general, and ways of communicating and counseling will be increasingly important for the profession. A service recommended by RDs who were surveyed in 2008[5] is a food and nutrition resource center in the ADA to assist dietitians working with ethnic groups.

Age Diversity

Baby Boomers are driving many of the health and nutrition practices today; however, both older and younger generations have ingrained attitudes that differ in some dramatic ways (Table 14-1). Fast-food preferences, image perceptions, and more of a tendency to turn to supplements for their nutrition concerns are among some of the characteristics of later generations.

Table 14-1. Generational Attitudes and Values Toward Food and Nutrition

Attitude/Value	Silent Generation (born before 1945)	Baby Boomers (born 1946–1964)	Generation X (born 1965–1985)	Gen Y (born 1986–present)
Attitudes to nutrition, health	Those aged 60–70 not silent and seeking more variety and more healthful choices. Have health concerns and interested in better diets.	A bit more active and exercise more. Trying to eat healthfully, more interested in nutrition, longevity.	More fast foods. Like supplements for health maintenance. May be uneducated about nutrition, but older Xers are getting the diet–health connection.	Want to know where the food comes from, how it was produced. Interested in organics.
Attitudes to nutrition, health	Don't want to waste food. Will exercise. Attribute health to moderate diet, daily activity, and not smoking.	Want to spend the second half of life healthy but over-ambitious in making changes.	Permissive parents, allow children to decide what to eat—kids can nag for favorite foods. Alternatively, pressure kids to be perfect.	Use supplements for the quick fix. The generation of artificial food stuffs, fast foods, with some exercise.
Attitudes to nutrition, health	Still have gardens, shop frugally, and know how to prepare, store food.	Have food skills, but financial freedom not to use. Some attracted to alternative medicines, others drug-reliant for health, mood.	Producing a generation of overweight children—high-energy snacks, little exercise. Interested in diet only when pregnant or caring for infants.	
Fads and new food habits	Eating out—we've earned it!	Acquired Starbucks habit, reverting to cocktails later in the day. Eating out or takeout because busy. Boomers always extremists.	Starbucks trendy drinks are the new cocktails for this generation. This is the fad diet generation. Sipping from water bottles all day. Confusion about carbohydrates and vegetarianism.	Sipping from water bottles all day. Restaurants are models for meals. Prefer eating out. Would prefer to drink their meals (e.g., supplements, fortified waters). Confusion about carbohydrates and vegetarianism.

Obsession with body image	Not a big concern.	High value: Self-absorbed and self-rationalizing: eating disorders kept secret, even from doctors and families.	High value: More open about eating disorders. Health less important than image.	High value: More open about eating disorders.
Changes in family life	Some experience with changes. Becoming more like Boomers in their family life.	Family meals rare and precious. Lack of time means quick food prep.	Many variations in family makeup, more single households. May not cook.	Norm: Everyone in the family operates individually. Can't cook, do not want to.
Approaches to life/work	Live to work, or did before they retired. Have had to learn the most: technologies, culture change, and so on.	Motivated by status, power, need for money to fund luxury lifestyles, work all hours.	Motivated by status, power, need for money to fund luxury lifestyles, work all hours. Less loyalty to employers, more turnover.	Less loyalty and desire to please employers. Expect autonomy and self-direction, high-status jobs, but overall, less driven.
Health: chronic problems	Need a diagnosis before acting.	More motivated to take charge of chronic conditions. Maybe half face heart attacks, diabetes, obesity.	More motivated to take charge of chronic conditions, and make changes before problems occur.	Want more information about chronic disease, learning about diabetes at a young age.
Educational strategies, concerns	Range from "too late to change now," to those with free time and interest in new strategies. Respectful and willing to listen.	Information NOW demanded. May be in denial and avoid learning. Older Boomers more willing to listen.	Willing to help with "causes" and be involved. Unsure of how to implement change. Information NOW demanded. Can be confrontational. Will pick and choose to suit what they want.	Needs entertainment to get the message. Wants information personalized—no groups! Information NOW demanded.

(continues)

Table 14-1. Generational Attitudes and Values Toward Food and Nutrition *(continued)*

Attitude/Value	Silent Generation (born before 1945)	Baby Boomers (born 1946–1964)	Generation X (born 1965–1985)	Gen Y (born 1986–present)
Dealing with growing older, diet, living, change, attitudes to the future	May be the last meat and potatoes generation. Will be slow, steady in change. Do what the doctor says, even when no longer relevant. Entitlement attitude may overwhelm social services/health care.	Still want center stage, won't be run off. Will want more ethnic influence and variety in assisted-living dining. More stress, seeking balance in busy lives, but question everything. "Live for the day" attitude, no concern for future health.	More questioning of the status quo and of authority. Want to negotiate change, prefer a quick fix, the magic pill, not to do the work. Are hardworking on their own terms, not including working on their own health, cooking meals, too busy. "Live for the day" attitude, no concern for future health. May become more concerned for their children's habits, health.	Invincibility of youth, unaware of long-term effects. Have heard the nutrition message in school—effect yet to be seen. Food an opportunity for casual contact, not long-term relationships. "It's not my problem" attitude. "Live for the day" attitude, no concern for future health.

Source: Jarrat, J. and J.B. Mahaffle. "The Profession of Dietetics at a Critical Juncture: A Report on the 2006 Environmental Scan for the American Dietetic Association." *J Am Diet Assoc* 107, no. 7(2007): 550–551.

Busy lifestyles and working family members have a tendency to lead to what is described as "fast-food, eat-and-run society." In turn, this leads to ever greater availability of fast food and ready-prepared food bought outside the home. Many young people grow up in homes where families do not eat together and do not learn cooking skills, leading to more permissiveness about food choices. Dietitians need to work with these trends, realizing that traditional approaches to counseling and food advising will have to change and adapt in order to face the realities of working with people of all ages and backgrounds. If the nutrition and health messages are to be effective, they must fit with consumer expectations.

Aging Population

The life expectancy in the United States has increased over the years, standing now at 77.7 years.[6] Better medical screening and treatment accounts for much of the advances along with lower death rates for some chronic diseases. While cardiovascular disease and cancer death rates have dropped, others such as Alzheimer's disease, kidney disease, hypertension, and Parkinson's disease are up. Further, obesity-related conditions are poised to increase in the future.[7]

The healthcare system is undergoing rapid change and one of the most significant aspects of this change is the increasing cost for chronic conditions affecting the aging population. Financial considerations may be a large factor in view of the fact that many lack health insurance and adequate access to health care. Preventive measures that focus on healthful lifestyle practices—nutrition being among the most important—will be increasingly needed. Dietitians will find more and varied opportunities in specialty areas of practice for the aging population, realizing that the needs of the elderly are often related to the presence of chronic conditions. People want to live as long and as well as they can and will benefit from healthful, helpful advice.

Health and Wellness

Because healthcare costs have a tremendous influence on the country's economy, we can expect the whole healthcare system to be reshaped in the future. The emphasis is likely to increasingly shift to disease prevention through exercise; employer incentive plans for employees regarding smoking, drugs, and the like; government policies that promote a healthful food supply; and consumer nutrition education. Dietitians are positioned to be in the forefront of many of these efforts.

Schools have an important role to play in overcoming the growing incidence of childhood obesity through physical education programs, school nutrition programs, and nutrition education. Without interventions now, whole generations may develop severe disease problems and early mortality. The ADA Foundation has named childhood obesity as a high priority area for both educational and funding efforts. School nutritionists can be leaders in these efforts.

Obesity among all age groups and even in many other countries of the world has worsened over the past 20 years and the Centers for Disease Control identify obesity as an epidemic with serious effects on public resources as well as health.[8] Identifying causes and finding more efficient and effective ways that lead to change are the challenges for dietitians along with all other health professions.

Communications

Communications Technology

The means of communication are continually evolving to the extent that computers, handheld devices, and cellular telephones are now commonplace in society. Electronic medical records are coming with implications for RDs in practice.[9] Social networks such as Facebook, LinkedIn, the ADA's Dietetics Community, and Foodservice-1 provide networking opportunities and facilitate the exchange of information with fellow professionals as well as other health groups and the public.[10]

An area of communication of great interest for its potential to healthcare providers is Telehealth. This is described as "the use of electronic information and telecommunications technologies to support long-distance clinical health care, patient and professional health-related education, public health, and health administration, and includes both the use of interactive, specialized equipment, for such purposes as health promotion, disease prevention, diagnoses, consultation, and/or therapy, and noninteractive (or passive) communications, over means such as the Internet, e-mail, or fax lines for communication of broad-based nutrition information that does not involve personalized nutrition recommendations or interventions."[11]

As is pointed out, this is as yet an unexplored area of communication and would have passive or interactive, interstate or intrastate, licensure, professional liability, privacy, and reimbursement issues to be resolved. Yet, dietitians need to be aware that this is a technology likely to receive more attention in the future and that practice will be greatly affected as a result.

Communicating

Informatics was discussed earlier as using and managing information, primarily by electronic means. The confidence the public has depends in great part on what is supplied by the media, therefore the need is great for the best information and dietitians are the primary source of valid information about nutrition.

Dietitians increasingly need to translate research findings that are sometimes confusing and contradictory. Media-savvy professionals can help with information about the latest fad diets, supplements, and alternative treatments that are often highly promoted by the media.[12] A "communication twilight zone" is described by Rowe and Alexander[13,14] in which anyone can broadly disseminate information today, with the result that dispute, argument, and conflict are sometimes the aim rather than solid, science-based information.

Environmental Issues

The trend toward "living green" is one that will continue to grow as more consumers turn to organic, locally grown foods and eco-friendly, household supplies. Organic foods and beverages are one of the fastest growing segments of the $598 billion food market today.[15] Reducing waste by recycling leads to significant reductions in environmental pollutants as well as overflowing landfills. Schools, healthcare, and commercial operations generate 35 to 45 percent of the total municipal solid waste in the United States[16] giving rise to the need for awareness and steps to handle waste items in more eco-friendly ways.

Other issues in environmental sustainability are energy and water consumption. Dietitians and those in commercial food establishments need to help select energy-saving equipment and take steps to reduce the amount of water used in food production. Examples of "going green" in hospitals are discussed in an issue of the *ADA Times,*[17] such as flexible menus in order to make the best use of foods in season, buying from local farmers and producers, and checking all processes for the best energy and water usage.

Even "greener" meetings need to be a goal of all professionals. This means meetings that minimize water and energy use, from the distance traveled to the meeting to the type and amount of food and water used, the energy used in lighting and electricity, the paper and plastic recycled, and the amount of waste left behind.[18]

Nutrigenomics and Nanotechnology

"Genetic dietetics" is a term becoming increasingly familiar as researchers publish rapidly developing findings about genetics. DeBusk[19–20] and others are alerting dietitians to the potential for individualized treatments and diets designed for each person's genetic makeup. A whole new field is evolving based on "nutrigenomics," or the scientific study of the way specific genes and bioactive food components interact.[21]

Genetic knowledge will be used in the future to avert childhood and adult obesity, metabolic syndrome, heart disease, and many other nutrition-related disorders. De Busk[22] points out that genetic information may well be a part of dietetics practice in the future and that standards of practice in regard to disclosure and privacy issues will be needed in working with patients.

Other "omics" are also being identified; namely, proteonomics and metabolomics (Figure 14-1). Kraswell[23] describes "epigenetics" and the way that environmental factors, such as food and supplement intake, can alter gene activity and thereby affect cellular function and metabolism. Practitioners with specialty training will be needed to conduct health as-

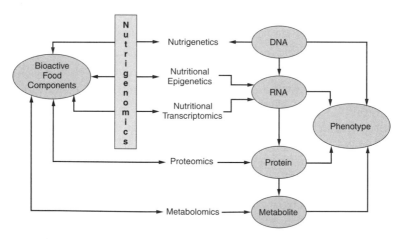

FIGURE 14-1. Nutritional "Omics."

Source: Trujllo, E., C. Davis, and J. Milner. "Nutrigenomics, Proteomics, Metabolomics, and the Practice of Dietetics." *J Am Diet Assoc* 106, no. 3(2006): 403–413.

sessments and counsel patients. Expansion of food composition data, new diagnostic tests, changes in the Dietary Reference Intakes (DRIs), and specialty foods are projected to occur in dietetics to support this new area.

Nanotechnology is another scientific breakthrough with exciting possibilities in dietetics practice.[24] New nutrient delivery systems, improvements in food safety and sanitation practices, and increases in the number of enriched and fortified food products may be possible with this new technology.

These new areas of science and research have profound implications for the dietetics profession, including continuing education as a crucial need. Positive attitudes are important but knowledge is essential for incorporating the new processes and procedures into practice.[25]

CHANGING ROLES IN THE HEALTHCARE SYSTEM

The early 1990s brought about fundamental changes in the American healthcare system. Mergers, consolidations, downsizing, and outsourcing transformed the entire way in which health services are delivered. New managed care and integrated health systems, organized along a complete continuum of care, replaced more traditional organizational structures. These systems were designed to respond to the need for cost reduction in the healthcare industry, to improve access to quality care, and to enhance client outcomes.

Along with challenges the dietetics profession faces as a result of the restructuring of the health industry, there are opportunities. Health care accounts for some 15 percent of the nation's gross domestic product.[26] The growth is driven by the Baby Boomers' desire to look and feel better and the elderly's desire to live longer. In particular, trend analysts predict continued growth in the diet and fitness industry.

Further good news for the profession is that in the market-driven healthcare delivery system, allied health professionals provide a cost-effective alternative to the more expensive services of physicians. To be competitive in new practice roles, allied health professionals will have to develop new roles and responsibilities. The Pew Health Professions Commission made strong recommendations about the competencies needed for these future roles: the ability to work in interdisciplinary teams; a reliance on health and information technologies strongly grounded in science and critical thinking; and cross-functional knowledge and skills.[27] The report also suggests the emergence of new allied health professions that will fall outside the sometimes rigid boundaries of currently recognized disciplines. This movement will require innovative approaches to role definition and partnership among allied health groups.

The profession's ability to continue to deliver high-quality, cost-effective care, to enter the curative and preventive market in low-cost settings, and to systematically document the impact of nutrition interventions will determine its future.

IMPLICATIONS AND CHALLENGES FOR THE PROFESSION

The value of describing a possible future for the profession is to be able to address the challenges faced by members of the profession and to take advantage of the opportunities the future offers. Although it is admittedly difficult to predict where the profession will be with such large changes, the questions to be asked are:

- What challenges will the future bring for the profession?
- What new assumptions will guide planning for the future of the profession?
- What new competencies will be needed by future professionals?

The dietetic profession faces a number of challenges as constantly changing events and trends inevitably shape practice.

The first challenge concerns positioning dietetic professionals in an industry characterized by changing health systems. Although dietitians have always focused on preventive care, they face intense competition from other healthcare providers, including those available via the Internet. Many health professionals are also struggling for recognition in these new health systems. The profession will need to deliver a new practitioner who brings both a multidisciplinary perspective and critical-thinking skills needed to solve both client and delivery-system problems.

The second challenge requires accepting the new world of work and redefining new practice roles. Future dietetic professionals will be entering a new world of work where practice will continually change. The turbulent healthcare marketplace continues to experience downsizing and dramatic restructuring, all of which affects the delivery of nutrition services. Fundamental changes will occur: jobs will evolve from being narrowly defined and task-oriented to more multidisciplinary and multidimensional roles; nothing will be permanent. Members of the profession will have to bring a generalist mindset to the practice area. Job flexibility will be a reality as professionals move in and out of careers and organizations many times throughout their lives.

The third challenge calls dietitians to keep the knowledge base current and obtain a commitment to lifelong learning. By definition, a professional is mandated to use the latest science in developing interventions and to keep practice standards current. With the rapid change in the knowledge that is brought to solve today's nutrition and eating problems, the issue of managing continuing professional education becomes a survival strategy. It has been suggested that half of what is learned as we enter the profession is obsolete within 3 years. This presents a tremendous need to develop lifelong learning models focusing on professional education.

The fourth challenge concerns education for the profession. New educational competencies for entry-level practice were issued in 2008. Earlier, an Education Task Force under the direction of the House of Delegates developed a far-reaching, future plan for dietetics education, which will carry the profession forward as it is implemented. Continuing education at advanced levels in order to absorb and apply constantly evolving new information needs to continue to be a major focus area for the profession. A form of competition that affects recognition and salaries for dietetics professionals is the comparison of education levels required for other professionals.[28] See Table 14-2.

The fifth challenge involves keeping pace with the reengineering occurring in the industries employing dietitians. Although most dietitians are employed in health care, there will continue to be a significant number employed in the food industry as well as in other developing industries. Like the healthcare industry, the food industry is experiencing downsizing, outsourcing, mergers, and acquisitions as a result of intense competition and downturns in the economy. These changes have major implications for food and nutrition specialists, some positive and others that could be destructive. Continual and overlapping change is occurring in industries and organizations in which dietetic professionals are employed, making it difficult to monitor trends shaping new practice roles.

Healthcare engineering is a trend with implications for dietitians as well.[29] The engineering profession has already introduced many new

Table 14-2. Entry-Level Education Requirements for Some Health Professions

Entry-Level Education Requirement	Health Professionals
Associate Degree	· Dietetic Technician, Registered · Respiratory Therapist—pursuing movement to a BS prepared clinician · Cardiovascular Technician · Registered Nurse (although there are many baccalaureate nursing degrees offered)
Baccalaureate Degree	· Registered Dietitian · Clinical Laboratory Technician · Radiology Technician—can also receive a certificate in training and/or associate degree
Advanced Degree	· Physical Therapist · Speech Pathologist · Occupational Therapist
Practice Doctorate	· PharmD · Audiologist · Dentist · Physician

Source: American Dietetic Association House of Delegates. "Dietetics Education and the Needs for the Future." *HOD Backgrounder,* 2003, pp. 1–2.

medical devices that have improved and extended the lives of millions. Artificial limbs, heart pacemakers, biosensors that detect nerve and muscle abnormalities, and robots that perform surgery are examples. The possibility of a digital interface with genomics and for information technology that can assist in personalized health care based on highly individualized information is further envisioned. Healthcare may look very different in the future, becoming more mechanized and individualized and leading to the need for all healthcare professionals to be informed and prepared to incorporate new procedures into practice.

The sixth challenge is continuing to strive for salary equity. The membership of the ADA, being predominantly female, faces societal trends that favor higher salaries for males in leadership roles. Even when controlling for gender differences in educational attainment, age, and experience, salary differentials continue to exist. According to the American College of Healthcare Executives, the median salaries for females as CEOs differ by almost $40,000 from males; among operating officers and vice presidents, salaries differ by about $25,000.[30] Weil and Mattis[31] offer recommendations for women in or aspiring to managerial and leadership roles as follows:

- Seek to work for organizations that are flexible.
- Avoid career interruptions of 6 months or more.
- Be willing to work whatever hours the job requires.
- Be willing to relocate if necessary.
- Aim for positions that are high in the organizational hierarchy.
- Stay focused on long-term goals.

Despite many challenges, the profession puts together an impressive number of winning combinations. Dietetics continues to be a highly respected profession, recognized worldwide as the leading organization of food and nutrition experts. With the aging population and the maturing Baby Boomers, the demand for dietetic professionals will increase. Additionally, the industry is already a generalist profession with the capability of easily moving into multidisciplinary and multifunctional careers. Finally, the profession has a long history of encouraging the growth and development of diversity.

The profession is likely to address these changes, in part, by restructuring itself around the technology of "connectivity" and in the way its members deliver services to consumers. If downsizing and outsourcing continue in both the healthcare and food industries, individuals will be working in small ad hoc work groups, taking on specific tasks, and then moving on to yet another work task. Relationships will not be permanent and employee–company loyalty will not be valued.

With continual and overlapping change in both practice settings and in interactions with others, what is brought to these new work groups will be cutting-edge knowledge and skills. To avoid obsolescence and to keep current with the search, learning and work will occur simultaneously. Technology-based, self-directed learning will occupy a large portion of the work day.

COMPETITION AND COLLABORATION WITH OTHER PROFESSIONS

Competition, driven by the information revolution, continues as entirely new professions and new competitive products and services emerge.

Virtual "meeting and dining" rooms allow consumers across the nation and around the world to meet without leaving home or work. More aging individuals can remain independent and in their own homes with the help of technological aids. Health organizations, linked electronically, provide access to experts around the world at the time the attending physician is in need of consultation. Digital highways provide immediate access to the world's retail marketplace for information, programs, services, and entertainment. Technology will change the nature of competition in ways one would never expect.

Probably the greatest "competitor" or "collaborator" is the rapid growth of information technology. It is the advent of the information age that is driving changes in business, government, professions, and social institutions. Future dietetic professionals will have a new set of leadership skills with a small specialty core of food, nutrition, and health. To compete, they will be experts at discovering, evaluating, and disseminating information and other resources. They will also need such futures-related leadership skills as visioning, persuasive communications, and the ability to form strategic partnerships.

COMPETENCIES OF THE FUTURE DIETETICS PROFESSIONAL

In his book, *The Knowledge Executive*, Cleveland[32] summarizes one of the most important critical skills of future professionals in the following statement: "People who do not educate themselves, and keep re-educating themselves, to participate in the new knowledge environment will be the peasants of the information society." Cleveland presents a strong case for not only understanding the power of being a "knowledge worker" in the 21st century but also for being technologically literate—being able to use existing or new technology to access and to manage the proliferation of knowledge. Others, within and outside the profession, also concur with the need for this competency.

There is general agreement among employers, educators, and practitioners that the following competencies will be needed in the future:[33]

> Leadership skills—Having the ability to see new opportunities, to create new visions for the profession, and to lead others through the milieu of change that will continue to be part of professional lives.

Professional and organizational awareness—Understanding the mission, vision, and goals of the dietetic profession; having the ability to link food and nutrition interventions to the overall health of the individual; seeing how nutrition care fits into the goals of employment sites; appreciating organizations as dynamic political, economic, and social systems.

Problem-definition and problem-solving skills—Identifying gaps between where a situation is and should be and helping others to see how to fill the gaps.

General business skills—Knowing the economic impacts of food and nutrition interventions; understanding strategic management, marketing, finance, logistics, accounting, and how these business functions work together.

Team-building and interpersonal skills—Having strong team-building skills because of the increasing use of outsourcing and temporary personnel; similarly, having persuasive communication skills to sell new ideas and to obtain support for change.

Entrepreneurialism—Having an ability to see new career opportunities; to combine that ability with necessary business skills; and to be a risk taker because of the shorter life cycles of most careers; implies a need to challenge traditional roles and prevailing approaches to delivering food and nutrition services.

Multicultural, multidiversity competence—Having an openness to other cultural values; a global understanding and perspective; and the attitudes, skills, and knowledge needed to apply a global perspective to clients, colleagues, and employees' needs.

FUTURE ROLES FOR THE PROFESSION

Opportunities in Health Care

The healthcare industry continues to grow and the cost of medical care for people over age 65 rises annually. The forces behind rising health costs are:[34]

- Advances in medical technology
- Aging
- Insufficient preventive care

- Rising government healthcare oversight and mandates
- Medicalization of more conditions
- Malpractice suits

Because of these trends, emphasis on preventive medicine is growing. Following this trend, the National Institutes of Health issues its "Healthy People" goals each decade that target specific disease conditions and environmental, societal, and communication needs toward improving the overall health of Americans.[35]

The demand for dietetic professionals is expected to grow as fast as the average for all industries in the nation's economy. There will be a need for increased meals and nutrition programs in long-term care, schools, correctional institutions, residential care, community health, home health care, and health and fitness clubs, to name a few. Traditional professional roles (such as food service administrator or clinical practitioner) will almost become obsolete in the future. The new healthcare environment will see dietetic professionals managing multiple departments or providing transdisciplinary health services, in which nutrition is only part of the practice role. In the future, it will not be uncommon to see food and nutrition experts earn dual degrees in medicine, pharmacy, nursing, physical therapy, law, or hotel and restaurant management.

Additionally, there will be some executive-level positions in integrated health systems and in traditional healthcare organizations. These positions will require a new set of competencies in such areas as strategic planning, information management, marketing, finance, and cost-benefit analysis.

Food

Large growth in employment for dietitians in the food and food service industries is anticipated as consumer food spending by 2017 approaches a trillion dollars a year.[36] Consumers want new foods and foods that are pure, natural, safe, and healthful. Convenience will continue to drive demand. Special food meals for segments of the population will also drive demand, especially the aging and those on weight-loss diets. The growing epidemic of obesity among children as well as adults means that dietitians with multiple backgrounds in food science, culinary arts, food product development, and exercise and fitness are and will continue to be in demand.

The commercial food service industry will continue to provide careers for those interested in combining an interest in foods, international cuisine, and business administration. Restaurant and in-home catering will grow as consumers entertain more and cook less. Resorts hire food professionals. Food manufacturers and food distributors look to members of the profession who can provide marketing support, sales training, new product development, and food photography support. Many hotels are setting up educational childcare centers for parents traveling with children; they need help with nutrition education programming, health and fitness programs, and developmentally appropriate feeding strategies. Associations representing health professions are also employing food and nutrition consultants to help develop transdisciplinary education programs.

Information Technology and Management

Varian[37] predicts more information specialists will be needed in the future "to rescue managers from the proliferation of knowledge" surrounding a profession. He suggests the following new career opportunities: organizers of user-friendly information on the Internet; database designers and managers; electronic writers and editors; instructional system designers; distance learning programmers and evaluators; and information entrepreneurs who can develop innovative ways for professionals and clients to connect and to work together. There will be a need for experts in such subspecialties as food and nutrition to develop, deliver, and evaluate these new and innovative educational programs. The information specialist, with a food and nutrition specialty, will be a critical future practitioner needed to organize and structure electronic data in a usable and easily accessible format.

Multimedia education and developing and selling electronic books, tapes, seminars, and speeches will be in demand. The amount of healthcare information accessible with information technology is increasing and the number of people with access to that information is growing. Households with a personal computer increased from 9.5 percent in 1984 to over 50 percent in 2002, and it is predicted that 70 percent of all households will own a computer by 2020.[38]

Research

With the advent of the information society, new opportunities will exist for those interested in the discovery of knowledge. There is a need for those interested in studying both nutrition science and nutrition intervention issues and problems. New and emerging clinical protocols, intervention trials, and cost-benefit studies must be tested. Genetics and biotechnology are driving the need for discovery as the effects on food and nutrition are being explored and the information made available to consumers. Similarly, there is a need for food researchers who want to develop new products or who want to understand consumer satisfaction and service quality factors. Marketing research also has tremendous growth potential as advances in the food delivery system must be modeled, simulated, and tested for quality, efficiency, cost-effectiveness, and consumer acceptance.

Public Service

Public service and the military offer expanding opportunities for the dietetics professional with many benefits and a range of activities. Military dietitians, for instance, fill a variety of roles today, from running healthcare facilities, stateside and abroad, to filling teaching and research positions, to creating health and wellness programs.[39] Over time, military RDs can move into management, such as hospital administration, one of the many opportunities for upward mobility.

Governmental agencies such as the U.S. Department of Agriculture and Health and Human Services, Congress, and governmental/industry associations such as the International Food Council employ dietitians. Others work in international food organizations such as the United Nations Food and Agriculture Organization (FAO). In these positions, they serve in policy development, consumer information, food and nutrition research, and school nutrition and food safety programs. Dietitians serve on the Dietary Goals and the MyPyramid planning groups. Others work for the Food and Nutrition Board of the National Academy of Sciences developing the DRIs.

These positions and others in public service offer opportunities that require innovation, motivation, and a willingness to set out on what can be quite different paths. Dietitians may well serve as lobbyists in the future and run for public office at every level of government.

Planning for the Future

In addressing the future, dietitians must meet the challenges brought about as a result of reengineering both the health delivery system and the food industry. Those individuals who can capitalize on future trends, who understand how basic assumptions will change dietetic practice, and who proactively search out new career opportunities will be well poised for the future. Others who naively believe the future is "more of the same" will find their positions disappearing—even after many years of dedicated service.

In analyzing the future, some things are certain—the profession must always expect the unexpected and assume the future is not an extension of the past. There are several assumptions that can be made about the future that will guide people in career decision making:

- The ability to connect electronically will continue to revolutionize how, when, and where dietetic professionals will practice.
- Professionals, not the organizations' management, will emerge as primary players in multidisciplinary teams; managers will become facilitators, coaches, and mentors.
- The concept of organization will expand to include links to all external partners, including consumers.
- Most people will be connected, worldwide, forming new professional opportunities and risks.
- Services and products that dietetic professionals offer to clients will be "informationalized"; databases will be built into most products, programs, and services offered to consumers.
- Competition will no longer be limited to local, regional, or national audiences; it will be worldwide.
- Continual and timely learning will be the rule for health providers and their clients.
- Most individuals will study and live with multiple cultures and languages.
- Professionals will become more entrepreneurial and innovative in their approach to career design.

As discussed, turbulent times create both opportunities and threats for members of the profession. How should individual members shape their careers to fit into future scenarios? Steps that can be taken now are:

- Be visionary and manage your own career. Make a conscious shift of mind not to rely on traditional practice roles. Be open to future opportunities.
- Build a portfolio of skills that will position you for future career changes. There will be a need for people who can increase productivity of resources and who can develop cost-effective solutions to problems.

- If you are not techno-literate, become so. Be able to design organizational and consumer programs that use multiple multimedia approaches and formats.
- Be adept at building relationships, both internal and external, to the profession. A distinct competitive advantage will come to those who know how to network and connect with consumers, experts, and information specialists.
- Become an expert at accessing, acquiring, disseminating, and evaluating knowledge. It is the key strategic resource.
- Consider working at the periphery of the profession and related professions and seek out new areas.
- The most critical skills that will be needed for success in the future include computer skills, statistical analyses, communication skills, an entrepreneurial outlook, financial management, critical analysis, strategic planning, negotiation, and motivation.

SUMMARY

The dietetic profession is changing and becoming increasingly responsive to the needs of consumers and the marketplace. Because of changes in population demographics, increasing globalization, and changes in the healthcare system, the profession is faced with unprecedented challenges, but also great opportunities. Planning toward and preparing for the future through developing technical and personal skills such as acquisition and dissemination of knowledge, leadership qualities, and willingness to change will serve the dietitian well into the future.

DEFINITIONS

Allied Health Professions. Healthcare organizations or groups providing services that supplement and assist those in direct health care.

Demographics. Population statistics relating to characteristics of those making up the population, such as births, deaths, and ages that are used in scientific studies.

Multicultural. A term referring to different cultures found in populations.

Multidisciplinary. Describing a collection of several disciplines either similar or diverse in nature.

REFERENCES

1. Parks, S.C. "The Future in Dietetics." In *Dietetics: Practice and Future Trends*. Aspen Publishers: Gaithersburg, MD; 1998, p. 311.

2. Booth, W. "One Nation, Indivisible: Is It History?" www.washingtonpost.com (Accessed November 15, 2009).

3. Perez-Escamilla, R. "Dietary Quality Among Latinos: Is Acculturation Making Us Sick?" *J Am Diet Assoc* 109, no. 6(2009): 988–991.

4. Ayala, G. X., Baquery, B., and Klinger, S. "A Systematic Review of the Relationship Between Acculturation and Diet Among Latinos in the United States: Implications for Future Research." *J Am Diet Assoc* 108, no. 8(2008): 1330–1334.

5. Rogers, D. "Report on the American Dietetic Association Commission on Dietetic Registration Needs Assessment." *J Am Diet Assoc* 109, no. 7(2009): 1283–1293.

6. Centers for Disease Control and Prevention. "Life Expectancy." www.cdc.gov/nchs (Accessed November 11, 2009).

7. Healthy People 2010. www.healthypeople.gov (Accessed October 20, 2009).

8. See Note 7.

9. Lane, M. "Streaming Soon to a Computer Near You: How Online Video Will Change Media (and Maybe Your Practice) Forever."*ADA Times* Sept/Oct (2007): 12–15.

10. Graham, L.K. "What Is Social Networking? And How Do I Get Clued in to LinkedIn?" *J Am Diet Assoc* 109, no. 1(2009): 184.

11. Busey, C. and P. Michael. "Telehealth—Opportunities and Pitfalls." *J Am Diet Assoc* 108, no. 8(2008): 1296–1301.

12. Brown, D. "Becoming a Media-Savvy Registered Dietitian." *J Am Diet Assoc* 106, no. 8(2006): 1163–1164.

13. Rowe, S. and N. Alexander. "Getting It Right in the Coming Communications Twilight Zone." *Nutr Today* 43, no. 5(2008): 217–220.

14. Rowe, S. and N. Alexander. "Communicating Dietary Guidelines to a Balking Public." *Nutr Today* 44, no. 2(2009): 81–84.

15. Cappellano, K.L. "Living Green." *Nutr Today* 44, no. 1(2009): 38–42.

16. Position Paper: "Position of the American Dietetic Association: Food and Nutrition Professionals Can Implement Practices to Conserve Natural Resources and Support Ecological Sustainability." *J Am Diet Assoc* 107, no. 6(2007): 1033–1043.

17. Mills, L.S. "From Local Chow to Green Machines: ADA Members Are Turning Foodservice into Eco-Friendly Operations." *ADA Times* Jan/Feb(2008): 12–16.

18. Arose, S. "A Guide to Greener Meetings." *J Am Diet Assoc* 109, no. 5(2009): 800–802.

19. DeBusk, R.M., C.P. Fogarty, J.M. Ordovas, and K.S. Kornman, "Nutritional Genomics in Practice. Where Do We Begin?" *J Am Diet Assoc* 105, no. 4(2005): 589–598.

20. DeBusk, R. "Diet-Related Disease, Nutritional Genomics, and Food and Nutrition Professionals." *J Am Diet Asssoc* 109, no. 3(2009): 410–413.

21. Trujllo, E., C. Davis, and J. Milner. "Nutrigenomics, Proteomics, Metabolomics, and the Practice of Dietetics." *J Am Diet Assoc* 106, no. 3(2006): 403–413.

22. Reilly, P.R. and R.M. DeBusk. "Ethical and Legal Issues in Nutritional Genomics." *J Am Diet Assoc* 108, no. 1(2008): 36–40.

23. Kraswell, G.P.A. "Epigenetics: How It Can Affect Dietetics Practice." *J Am Diet Assoc* 108, no. 7(2008): 1056–1059.

24. Nickols-Richardson, S.M. "Nanotechnology: Implications for Food and Nutrition Professionals." *J Am Diet Assoc* 107, no. 9(2007): 1494–1497.

25. Rosen, R., C. Earthman, L. Marquart, and M. Reicka. "Continuing Education Needs of Registered Dietitians Regarding Nutrigenomics." *J Am Diet Assoc* 106, no. 8(2006): 1242–1245.

26. *Health and Health Care 2010: The Institute for the Future.* Jossey-Bass Co.: San Francisco; 2000.

27. Pew Health Professions Commission. *Critical Challenges: Revitalizing the Health Professions for the Twenty-First Century.* U.F.S.S. Center for Health Professions: San Francisco; 1995.

28. American Dietetic Association House of Delegates. "Dietetics Education and the Needs for the Future." *HOD Backgrounder* (2003).

29. Noor, A. "Re-engineering Health Care." *Mechanical Engineering* 129, no. 11(2007): 22–27.

30. Lantz, P.M. "Gender and Leadership in Healthcare Administration: 21st Century Progress and Challenges." *J Healthcare Management* 53(2008): 291–303.

31. Weil, P.A. and M.C. Mattis. "Narrowing the Gender Gap in Healthcare Management." *Healthcare Executive* 16, no. 6(2001): 12–17.

32. Cleveland, H. *The Knowledge Executive.* Truman Talley Books/EP Dutton: New York; 1989.

33. See Note 1.

34. House of Delegates Report. "Key Trends Affecting the Dietetics Profession and the American Dietetic Association. *J Am Diet Assoc* 102, no. 12(2002): S1821–1839.

35. Office of Disease Prevention and Health Promotion. "Healthy People 2010." www.healthypeople.gov/data/midcourse/html/execsummary/introduction.htm. U.S. Department of Health and Human Services (Accessed September 12, 2008).

36. See Note 1.

37. Varian, H. "The Next Generation Information Manager." *Educom Review* (1997): 12–14.

38. See Note 28.

39. Mathieu, J. "RDs in the Military." *J Am Diet Assoc* 108, no. 12(2008): 1984–1987.

Code of Ethics for the Profession of Dietetics and Process for Consideration of Ethics Issues (2009)

PREAMBLE

The American Dietetic Association (ADA) and its credentialing agency, the Commission on Dietetic Registration (CDR), believe it is in the best interest of the profession and the public it serves to have a Code of Ethics in place that provides guidance to dietetic practitioners in their professional practice and conduct. Dietetics practitioners have voluntarily adopted this Code of Ethics to reflect the values and ethical principles guiding the dietetics profession and to set forth commitments and obligations of the dietetics practitioner to the public, clients, the profession, colleagues, and other professionals. The current Code of Ethics was approved on June 2, 2009, by the ADA Board of Directors, House of Delegates, and the Commission on Dietetic Registration.

APPLICATION

The Code of Ethics applies to the following practitioners:

(a) In its entirety to members of ADA who are Registered Dietitians or Dietetic Technicians.

(b) Except for sections dealing solely with the credential, to all members of ADA who are not RDs or DTRs; and

(c) Except for aspects dealing solely with membership, to all RDs and DTRs who are not members of ADA.

FUNDAMENTAL PRINCIPLES

1. The dietetics practitioner conducts himself/herself with honesty, integrity, and fairness.

2. The dietetics practitioner supports and promotes high standards of professional practice. The dietetics practitioner accepts the obligation to protect clients, the public, and the profession by upholding the Code of Ethics for the profession of Dietetics and by reporting perceived violations of the Code through the processes established by ADA and its credentialing agency, CDR.

3. The dietetics practitioner considers the health, safety, and welfare of the public at all times.

4. The dietetics practitioner complies with all laws and regulations applicable or related to the profession or to the practitioner's ethical obligations as described in this Code.

5. The dietetics practitioner provides professional services with objectivity and with respect for the unique needs and values of individuals.

6. The dietetics practitioner does not engage in false or misleading practices or communications.

7. The dietetics practitioner withdraws from professional practice when unable to fulfill his or her professional duties and responsibilities to clients and others.

8. The dietetics practitioner recognizes and exercises professional judgment within the limits of his or her qualifications and collaborates with others, seeks counsel, or makes referrals as appropriate.

9. The dietetics practitioner treats clients and patients with respect and consideration.

10. The dietetics practitioner protects confidential information and makes full disclosure about any limitations on his or her ability to guarantee full confidentiality.

11. The dietetics practitioner, in dealing with and providing services to clients and others, complies with the same principles set forth above.

12. The dietetics practitioner practices dietetics based on evidence-based principles and current information.

13. The dietetics practitioner presents reliable and substantiated information and interprets controversial information without personal bias, recognizing that legitimate differences of opinion exist.

14. The dietetics practitioner assumes a life-long responsibility and accountability for personal competence in practice, consistent with accepted professional standards, continually striving to increase professional knowledge and skills and to apply them in practice.

15. The dietetics practitioner is alert to the occurrence of a real or potential conflict of interest and takes appropriate action whenever a conflict arises.

16. The dietetics practitioner permits the use of his or her name for the purpose of certifying that dietetics services have been rendered only if he or she has provided or supervised the provision of those services.

17. The dietetics practitioner accurately presents professional qualifications and credentials.

18. The dietetics practitioner does not invite, accept, or offer gifts, monetary incentives, or other considerations that affect or reasonably give an appearance of affecting his/her professional judgment.

19. The dietetics practitioner demonstrates respect for the values, rights, knowledge, and skills of colleagues and other professionals.

Adapted from: "The American Dietetic Association/Commission on Dietetic Registration Code of Ethics for the Profession of Dietetics and Process for Consideration of Ethics Issues." *J Am Diet Assoc* 109, no. 8(2009): 1461–1467.

Article II of the Bylaws of the American Dietetic Association

MEMBERS

Section 1. Classes of Members. The Association shall have the following five (5) classes of members:

Active   Retired   Student   Honorary   International

Section 2. Active Members. Qualifications.

2a. An individual holding a baccalaureate degree from a regionally accredited college or university, and meeting the academic requirements specified by the Association, plus one or more of the following criteria may apply for Active membership:

1. a Registered Dietitian ("RD") credentialed by the Commission on Dietetic Registration ("CDR");
2. completed an academic and/or supervised practice program accredited by the Commission on Accreditation for Dietetics Education ("CADE").

2b. An individual holding a master's or a doctoral degree, and a degree (baccalaureate, master's, doctoral) in one of the following areas may apply for Active membership: dietetics, foods and nutrition, nutrition, community/public health nutrition, food science, or food service systems management. A regionally accredited college or university must have conferred each degree.

253

    2c. An individual meeting one or more of the following criteria may apply for Active membership:
1. a Dietetic Technician, Registered ("DTR") credentialed by the CDR or has established eligibility to take the examination for dietetic technicians;
2. completed a CADE-approved associate degree program for dietetic technicians;
3. holds a baccalaureate degree and meets the academic requirements specified by CADE, and has completed a CADE accredited/ approved dietetic technician program experience.

    2d. An individual who previously paid the optional one-time dues in order to obtain "life" membership in the Association, or has completed a term as President of the Association.

Section 3. Retired Members. Qualifications. Any dietetics professional qualifying for the Active membership category that is no longer employed in dietetic practice or education and is at least sixty-two (62) years of age, or is retired on total (permanent) disability may apply for Retired membership.

Section 4. Student Members. Qualifications. Student classification can be held for a maximum of six (6) years. An individual meeting one of the following criteria may apply for Student membership:

    4a. A student enrolled in a CADE-accredited/approved program;

    4b. A student in a regionally accredited college or university who states his/her intent to enter a CADE-accredited/approved program;

    4c. Active members returning to school on a full-time basis for a baccalaureate or graduate degree in a dietetic-related course of study may apply for Student membership status.

Section 5. Honorary Members. Qualifications. An individual who has made a notable contribution to the field of nutrition and dietetics may be admitted to the Association as an Honorary member upon invitation of the Board of Directors.

Section 6. International Members. Qualifications. An individual who has completed formal training in food, nutrition, or dietetics outside the United States and U.S. Territories verified by the country's professional dietetics association and/or country's regulatory body.

Section 7. Privileges of Membership.

7a. Active Members. Active members whose dues are not in arrears shall be entitled one vote in each matter submitted to vote of members and are eligible to hold elected and appointed offices and positions at the national level. Active members shall be eligible to hold elected and appointed offices and positions at the affiliate level as designated by the affiliate dietetic association.

7b. Retired Members. Retired members whose dues are not in arrears shall be entitled to all the rights of the Active membership category.

7c. Student Members. Student members whose dues are not in arrears shall have the right to vote in the national and affiliate elections and are eligible to hold appointed positions at the national and affiliate levels if a resident of the U.S. or U.S. Territories. Student members shall not have a right to hold elected positions on the national and affiliate levels.

7d. Honorary Members. Honorary members may serve as members of committees and attend meetings. Honorary members shall not be entitled to vote or eligible to hold elected office.

7e. International Members. International members may be members of committees and attend meetings. International members shall be entitled to vote and eligible to hold elected office at the affiliate level.

7f. Voting. Each member eligible to vote shall be entitled to one vote on each matter submitted to a vote of the members.

Section 8. Termination and Reinstatement of Membership. The Board of Directors or its designee may terminate a member in default in the payment of dues. The House of Delegates ("HOD") or its designee may terminate membership for cause. Any former member who forfeited membership for nonpayment of dues may be reinstated to their former classification by paying the current annual dues and a reinstatement fee, and meeting the association's reinstatement requirements. Former members from the retired and returning student classes will be reinstated into the active class. Any former member whose membership was terminated for cause may request reinstatement of membership following one (1) year of termination unless otherwise determined by the HOD.

Source: American Dietetic Association. "Bylaws of the American Dietetic Association." 2008.

Headquarters
Organization Chart

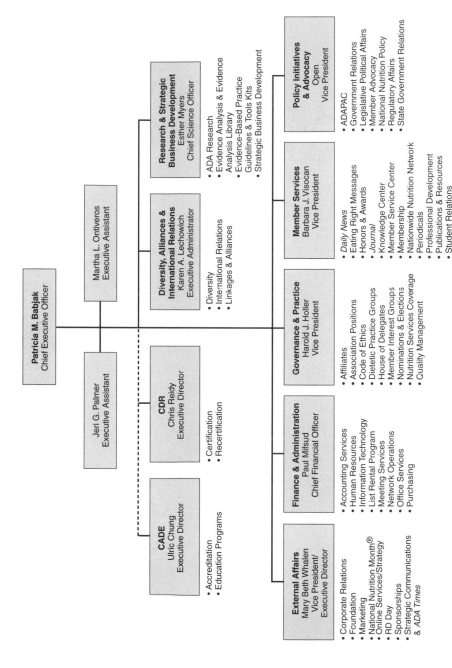

Source: American Dietetic Association.

Sub-Units of Dietetic Practice Groups and Member Interest Groups

DIETETIC PRACTICE GROUP SUB-UNITS

A dietetic practice group (DPG) may develop recognized sub-units or groups of members within the DPG based on a practice area or issue of interest to the members of the DPG. Currently over 30 of these sub-specialty areas exist within the main DPGs. The current list is as follows:

Name of Sub-Unit	DPG Affiliation
Food and Nutrition Informatics	CNM
Home Care	DHCC
Corrections	DHCC
Food Safety	FCP
Restaurant and Retail Foodservice	FCP
Supermarket	FCP
Dietitians in Gluten Intolerance Disease	MNPG
Dietitians in Physical Medicine and Rehabilitation	MNPG

(continues)

Name of Sub-Unit	DPG Affiliation
Authors	NE
Private Practice	NE
Corporate Health	NE
Internet	NE
Speakers	NE
Health Coaches	NE
Research	ONDPG
Complementary Nutrition	ONDPG
Hospice and Palliative Care	ONDPG
Pediatric Oncology	ONDPG
Cancer Prevention	ONDPG
Survivorship	ONDPG
Children with Special Health Care Needs	PNPG
Infant Nutrition/Breastfeeding with Neonatology	PNPG
Diabetes with Wellness and Weight Management	PNPG
Gastroenterology/Food Allergy with Failure to Thrive	PNPG
Nutrition Support	PNPG
Eating Disorder/Adolescents	PNPG
Clinical and Translational Science	RDPG
Disordered Eating	SCAN
CV-Wellness	SCAN
Sports Dietetics USA	SCAN
Bariatrics	WM
Pediatric Weight Management	WM

MEMBER INTEREST GROUPS (MIGs) 2008–2009

Chinese American in Dietetics and Nutrition (CADN)
CADN is the advocate of the dietetic profession serving those who are interested in the betterment of the nutritional needs of the Chinese. By promoting optimal use of research, presentations, and dissemination of literature, we work to enhance the nutritional status of Chinese in the United States and worldwide.

Filipino Americans in Dietetics and Nutrition (FADAN)
FADAN fosters a networking, mentoring, and support system that is sensitive to the professional issues unique to the Filipino-American dietitians, focusing on the diversity and ethnicity of this population.

Fifty Plus in Nutrition and Dietetics (FPIND)
The Fifty Plus in Nutrition and Dietetics MIG will focus on programming and networking targeted at members age 50 and older. In addition, this group will provide education and networking opportunities for those re-entering the workforce toward changing their career focus.

Latinos and Hispanics in Dietetics and Nutrition (LAHIDAN)
Fostering the development and improvement of food, nutrition, and health care for Latinos and their families in U.S. and related territories with outreach to Hispanics/Latinos and all other ADA members.

National Organization of Blacks in Dietetics and Nutrition (NOBIDAN)
The National Organization of Blacks in Dietetics and Nutrition is an organization of African-American Dietetic and Nutrition Practitioners whose mission is to develop an innovative plan with futuristic vision and ideals that will reflect concern for health status of the public and facilitate professional enhancement for its members.

National Organization of Men in Nutrition (NOMIN)
In conjunction with the ADA, the National Organization of Men in Nutrition values and respects the diverse viewpoints and individual differences of all people. Our mission and goal is to promote dietetics careers to all males and to support men who are nutritionists or DTRs to grow professionally.

Source: Courtesy of the American Dietetic Association. Dietetic Practice Group Sub-Units. http://webrd.org/cps/rde/xchg/ada/hs.xsl/career_485_ENU_HTML.htm. Accessed December 4, 2009.

Position Paper Update for 2009

FOOD CHOICES

- Total diet approach to communicating food and nutrition information. *J Am Diet Assoc.* 2007;107:1224–1232. (Expires 2011)
- Vegetarian diets. *J Am Diet Assoc.* 2003;103:748–765. ADA and Dietitians of Canada Joint Position. (Reaffirmed, updated position to be published in 2009)
- Health implications of dietary fiber. *J Am Diet Assoc.* 2008;108: 1716–1731. (Expires 2013)
- Functional foods. *J Am Diet Assoc.* 2004;204:814–826. (Reaffirmed, updated position to be published in 2009)
- Dietary fatty acids. *J Am Diet Assoc.* 2007;107:1599–1611. (Expires in 2009)

FOOD SUPPLY

- Safety
  Food and water safety. *J Am Diet Assoc.* 2003;103:1203. (Reaffirmed, updated position to be published in 2009)
- Supplementation/Fortification
  The impact of fluoride on health. *J Am Diet Assoc.* 2005;105: 1620–1628. (Reaffirmed, updated position to be published in 2010)

Fortification and nutritional supplements. *J Am Diet Assoc.* 2005; 105:1300–1311. (Reaffirmed, updated position to be published in 2009)

- Substitutes

Use of nutritive and nonnutritive sweeteners. *J Am Diet Assoc.* 2004; 104:255–275. (Reaffirmed, updated position to be published in 2010)

- Food Security/Environment

Agricultural and food biotechnology. *J Am Diet Assoc.* 2006;106: 285–293. (Expires 2010)

Food insecurity and hunger in the US. *J Am Diet Assoc.* 2006; 106:446–458. (Reaffirmed, updated position to be published in 2009)

Food and nutritional professionals can implement practices to conserve natural resources and protect the environment. *J Am Diet Assoc.* 2007;107:1033–1043. (Expires 2010)

Addressing world hunger, malnutrition, and food insecurity. *J Am Diet Assoc.* 2003;103:1046. (Reaffirmed, updated position to be published in 2009)

LIFE SPAN

- Pregnancy/Breastfeeding

Promoting and supporting breastfeeding. *J Am Diet Assoc.* 2005; 105:810–818. (Reaffirmed, updated position to be published in 2009)

Nutrition and lifestyle for a healthy pregnancy outcome. *J Am Diet Assoc.* 2008;108:553–561 (Expires 2011)

- Infancy/Childhood

Child and adolescent food and nutrition programs. *J Am Diet Assoc.* 2006;106:1467–1475. (Reaffirmed, updated position to be published in 2009)

Dietary guidance for healthy children ages 2–11 years. *J Am Diet Assoc.* 2008;108:1038–1047. (Expires 2011)

Local support for nutrition integrity in schools. *J Am Diet Assoc.* 2006;106:122–133. (Reaffirmed, updated position to be published in 2009)

Benchmarks for nutrition programs in child care settings. *J Am Diet Assoc.* 2005;105:979–986. (Reaffirmed, updated position will be published in 2009)

Nutrition services: An essential component of comprehensive school health programs. *J Am Diet Assoc.* 2003;102:505. (Reaffirmed, updated position to be published in 2009) ADA, American School Food Service Association and Society for Nutrition Education Joint Position

- Adults

Nutrition and athletic performance for adults. *J Am Diet Assoc.* 2000; 100:1543. (Reaffirmed, updated position to be published in 2009) ADA, Dietitians of Canada and American College of Sports Medicine Joint Position

- Older Adults

Liberalization of the diet prescription improves quality of life for older adults in long-term care. *J Am Diet Assoc.* 2005;106: 1955–1965. (Reaffirmed, updated position to be published in 2010)

Nutrition across the spectrum of aging. *J Am Diet Assoc.* 2005;105: 616–633. (Reaffirmed, updated position to be published in 2009)

NUTRITION MANAGEMENT

- Disease/Special Conditions

Nutrition intervention in the treatment of anorexia nervosa, bulimia nervosa, and other eating disorders. *J Am Diet Assoc.* 2006;106: 2073–2082. (Expires 2010)

Nutrition intervention in the care of persons with human immunodeficiency virus infection. *J Am Diet Assoc.* 2004;104:1425–1441. (Reaffirmed, updated position to be published in 2009) ADA and Dietitians of Canada Joint Position

Providing nutrition services for infants, children, and adults with developmental disabilities and special health care needs. *J Am Diet Assoc.* 2004;104:97–107. (Reaffirmed, updated position to be published in 2009)

Ethical and legal issues in nutrition, hydration, and feeding. *J Am Diet Assoc.* 2008;873–882. (Expires 2011)

- MNT/Health Care

  Integration of medical nutrition therapy and pharmacotherapy. *J Am Diet Assoc.* 2003;103:1363. (Reaffirmed, updated position to be published in 2009)

- Weight Management

  Weight management. *J Am Diet Assoc.* 2002;102:1145. (Reaffirmed, updated position to be published in 2009)

  Individual-, family-, school-, and community-based interventions for pediatric overweight. *J Am Diet Assoc.* 2006;106:925–945. (Expires 2010)

- Public Health

  Oral health and nutrition. *J Am Diet Assoc.* 2007;107:1418–1428. (Expires 2010)

  The roles of registered dietitians and dietetic technicians, registered in health promotion and disease prevention. *J Am Diet Assoc.* 2006;106:1875–1884. (Expires 2009; will be developed into a practice paper)

  Food and nutrition misinformation. *J Am Diet Assoc.* 2006;106:601–607. (Expires 2010)

POSITIONS TO EXPIRE DECEMBER 31, 2008

- Addressing world hunger, malnutrition, and food insecurity
- Benchmarks for nutrition programs in childcare settings
- Fat replacers
- Fortification and nutritional supplements
- Nutrition intervention in the care of persons with human immuno-deficiency virus infection
- Nutrition services: An essential component of comprehensive school health programs
- Promoting and supporting breastfeeding
- Providing nutrition services for infants, children, and adults with developmental disabilities and special healthcare needs
- Nutrition and women's health

POSITION PAPERS PUBLISHED IN 2009

- Position of the American Dietetic Association. "Functional Foods." *J Am Diet Assoc* 109, no. 4(2009): 735–746.

- Position of the American Dietetic Association and American Society for Nutrition. "Obesity, Reproduction, and Pregnancy Outcomes." *J Am Diet Assoc* 109, no. 5(2009): 918–927.
- Position of the American Dietetic Association. "Vegetarian Diets." *J Am Diet Assoc* 109, no. 7(2009): 1266–1282.

Source: American Dietetic Association. "Position Paper Update for 2009." *J Am Diet Assoc* 109, no. 2(2009): 347–348.

Index

Figures and tables are indicated by f and t following the page number.

A

AAFCS (American Association for Families and Consumer Sciences), 14
Academic health centers, 160, 217–218, 220
Accessibility of health care, 226
Accreditation, 38–39, 48. *See also* Commission on Accreditation for Dietetics Education (CADE); Credentialing
ADA House of Delegates and, 26
defined, 48
Didactic Program in Dietetics, 38–39, 40–41, 48, 57
Dietetic Technician Program, 11, 41, 44, 57–58
"Foundation Knowledge and Competencies" (CADE), 40
of hospitals, 14
of supervised practice programs, 43
Acute care
cardiac rehabilitation programs in, 151
clinical practice in, 11, 87, 95, 100
food and nutrition management in, 105–106
ADA. *See* American Dietetic Association
ADAF. *See* American Dietetic Association Foundation
Adherence counseling skills, 188
Administration, 7, 11, 52. *See also* Food and nutrition systems management

Adolescents
attitudes toward food and nutrition, 227, 228–230*t*
disordered eating in, 153–154
fitness centers for, 150
obesity in, 148
school-based health centers for, 155
Adult health promotion specialists, 122
Adults
attitudes toward food and nutrition, 227, 228–230*t*
health problems associated with diets of, 147
health promotions for, 120, 122–124
as learners, 205–206
obesity of, 148
Adult Weight Management Certificate of Training, 59–60
Advanced-level education. *See* Continuing education; Graduate education
Advanced-levels of practice, 59. *See also* Specialties of practice
Age diversity, 174, 227, 228–230*t*, 231
Aging population, 152, 203*f*, 204, 226–227, 228–230*t*, 231, 240
Agriculture Department, U.S. (USDA), 78
Alliance for a Healthier Generation, 16
Allied health professions, 157, 235, 236, 237, 238*t*, 246
Ambulatory care, 87, 94

American Association for Families and
   Consumer Sciences (AAFCS), 14
American College of Healthcare Executives,
   238–239
American College of Sports Medicine
   Exercise Test Technology certification,
   139
American Diabetes Association, 14
American Dietetic Association (ADA),
   19–33
   ADAF. *See* American Dietetic Association
      Foundation
   affiliated units, 31–32
   benefits, 22
   Board of Directors (BOD), 24–25
   bylaws, 20, 33, 253–255
   CADE. *See* Commission on Accreditation
      for Dietetics Education
   CDR. *See* Commission on Dietetic
      Registration
   Center for Professional Development, 69
   Center for Professional Education, 9, 69
   chief executive officer, 24, 33
   contact information, 15
   DPGs. *See* Dietetic Practice Groups
   ethics. *See* "Code of Ethics for the
      Profession of Dietetics and the Process
      for Consideration of Ethics Issues
      (2009)"
   founding of, 6–7
   governance of, 24–31, 25*f,* 33, 258
   history of, 6–8
   House of Delegates (HOD), 25–26, 42
   legislative activity, 11, 32, 78
   logo, 21
   long-range planning, 12–13
   membership, 9–10, 24, 43, 47, 52
   membership benefits, 22
   membership categories, 21–22, 47,
      253–255
   MIGs. *See* Member Interest Groups
   mission statement, 20
   political action committee, 11
   position papers. *See* Position papers
   publications, 43, 47, 233
   public outreach, 9, 13, 15–16, 52
   public policy, 78, 79
   registration, 10, 13, 27, 53, 54, 57–58,
      61
   Research Committee, 213–215
   research philosophy of, 213
   social networks of, 232
   state and district associations, 31
   strategic plan, 13, 20–21, 33
   Task Forces, 13, 42, 56, 98–99
   trends study, 42–43
   values, 20, 67
   Washington office, 11, 32
American Dietetic Association Foundation
   (ADAF), 10, 21, 24, 31–32, 232
American Home Economics Association, 6,
   14
American Hospital Association, 14
American Overseas Dietetic Association
   (AODA), 15
American Public Health Association
   (APHA), 14
American Red Cross, 5, 6
AMFO (Association for Managers of Food
   Operations), 10–11
Amines, 4
Anorexia nervosa, 153–154, 161
Areas of practice, 7, 11–12, 12*t*
   in business and communications,
      144–146
   in cardiovascular nutrition, 151
   in clinical nutrition, 87, 87*t,* 88*t,* 95
   in community and public health, 118,
      120, 122–124, 123*t*
   as consultants, 132, 134–135, 137–138,
      137–139*t*
   for DTRs, 55–57
   in food and food service, 242–243
   in food companies, 218
   in for-profit businesses, 144
   future, 236–237, 241–244
   in government centers and laboratories,
      218–219
   history of, 7
   in industry, 218
   in information technology, 243
   in research, 158–159, 217–220
   in sports nutrition, 149–150
   in wellness and health promotion, 148,
      151–152
Assessment
   in community and public health
      nutrition, 125

defined, 140, 208
in food services, 133
instruments for, 191–192
of needs of learners, 189
in nutrition care process and model, 90, 93, 97
in standards of practice, 93
Assistants, dietetic, 98
Association for Managers of Food Operations (AMFO), 10–11
Asynchronous technologies in distance learning, 71
Athletic performance and nutrition, 148–149
Attitudes toward food and nutrition, 227, 228–230*t*

B
Baby Boomers, 227, 228–230*t*, 239
Barber, Mary E., 8
Beach, Anna Boller, 8
Behavioral and social science research, 214
Behavioral learning, 188
Benchmarking, 176, 182
Binge eating disorders, 153–154, 161
Board of Directors (ADA), 24–25
Bryan, Mary deGarmo, 8
Bulimia nervosa, 153–154, 161
Business and communications, 144–147, 145*t*
Business and consultation nutrition, 11, 12*t*, 22–24, 23*t*. *See also* Business and communications; Consultants
Business practice consultants, 134–135
Business skills, 241
Bylaws (ADA), 20, 33, 253–255

C
California mentoring program, 196–197
Cancer, 147–148
Carbohydrates, 4
Cardiac rehabilitation, 151
Cardiovascular disease, 147–148
Cardiovascular nutrition, 151, 161
Career opportunities. *See* Areas of practice
Career paths
    for business and communications dietitians, 144

for community nutrition dietitians, 122–124, 123*t*
for dietitians, 112
DTR registration eligibility pathway, 56, 57–58
in food and nutrition systems management, 108, 112–113, 242–243
"Future Practice and Education" Task Force, 13, 42, 53
Carry the Flame: The History of the American Dietetic Association (Cassell), 8
CDR. *See* Commission on Dietetic Registration
Center for Professional Development (ADA), 69. *See also* Professional development
Center for Professional Education (ADA), 9, 69. *See also* Education of dietetic professional
Centers for Disease Control, 232
Centers for Medicare and Medicaid Services (CMS), 131
Certificates of Training, 59–60
Certification, 63, 70–71. *See also* Credentialing; Licensure; Registration
    by AMFO, 10–11
    CDR. *See* Commission on Dietetic Registration
    Certificates of Training, 59–60
    development of, 53
    DTR certification, 57
    DTR recertification, 57, 60
    "Fellow of the American Dietetic Association," 59
    other health professions, 139
    RD certification, 10, 53–54
    RD recertification, 54, 57, 60
    specialist certification, 59, 60, 69
    specialist recertification, 60–61
    by states, 61–62
Certified food managers, 11
Change management, 179–180
Changing roles in healthcare systems, 235–236
Chief clinical dietitians, 94. *See also* Management
Chief executive officer (ADA), 24, 33

Childhood and Adolescent Weight
    Management Certificate of Training,
    59–60
Children
    attitudes toward food and nutrition, 227,
        228–230*t*
    childhood obesity, 16, 148, 150, 153, 232
    developmental diseases, 122–123
    fast food, 227
    fitness centers for, 150
    maternal and child health, 11, 123
    nutrition education in schools, 155
    school nutrition, 11, 107–108
    WIC, 78, 120
Chronic dieting, 153–154
Chronic diseases, 119, 122, 124, 147–148,
    231. *See also specific diseases*
Civil War, 6
Client, defined, 125, 140
Client-based focus in public health, 118,
    120, 124, 125
Client-centered counseling, 198
Clinical dietetics, defined, 101
Clinical Laboratory Improvement
    Certification, 139
Clinical nutrition, 7, 85–102
    acute and ambulatory care in, 11, 95, 100
    areas of practice, 11, 12*t*
    chief clinical dietitian, 94
    clinical dietitians, 94–95, 96–97*t*
    clinical privileging, 100
    communication methods, 99–100
    dietetic assistants, 98
    dietetic technicians, 56, 95–98
    employment settings, 86–88, 87*t*, 88*t*
    evidence analysis process in, 215–217,
        216*f*
    evidence-based practice in, 75–76,
        76–77*t*
    healthcare reform and, 98–99
    inpatient care, 108, 128
    managers, 88, 94, 108
    medical nutrition therapy, 7, 32, 92–93,
        98, 101, 130–131
    nutrition care process and model, 90–92,
        91*f*, 93–94
    organization of services in, 88–89, 89*f*
    public opinion survey on, 99
    research applications in, 215–217, 216*f*
    responsibilities in, 90–94, 96–97*t*
    service teams, 88, 89*f*, 94–98
    sports nutritionist, clinical concerns of,
        149, 149*t*
    standards of practice, 93–94
    supervised practice in, 43
Clinical Nutrition Management (DPG), 94
Clinical privileging, 99–100
CMS (Centers for Medicare and Medicaid
    Services), 131
Coaching, 174–175, 182, 197. *See also*
    Mentoring
"Code of Ethics for the Profession of
    Dietetics and the Process for
    Consideration of Ethics Issues (2009),"
    9, 57, 69, 249–251
Cognitive interviewing, 198
Cognitive learning, 188
Cognitive skills, 190, 208
Colleges and universities, 107, 156,
    217–218. *See also* Education of dietetic
    professional; Graduate education
Commercial food services, 107, 108–109,
    242–243. *See also* Food and nutrition
    systems management
Commission on Accreditation for Dietetics
    Education (CADE), 26–27. *See also*
    Accreditation
    Dietetic Technician Program, 41
    "Foundation Knowledge and
        Competencies," 40
    logo, 21
    program requirements, 38–39
Commission on Dietetic Registration
    (CDR), 27, 54, 57–58, 61, 187. *See*
    also Credentialing; Registration
Communication
    clinical practice, 99–100
    educators as communicators, 202–204,
        202*f*, 203*f*
    skills in management, 174, 180
    standards of professional practice, 109
    technology, 232–233
*Communication and Education Skills: The
    Dietitian's Guide* (Holli & Calabrese),
    174
Communication and media specialists, 123

Community, defined, 125
Community and public health nutrition, 7,
    11, 12*t*, 117–126
    activities of community dietitians,
        120–122
    areas of practice, 118, 120, 122–124
    career outlook, 124
    career paths, 122–124, 123*t*
    community assessment, defined, 125
    community health services, defined, 125
    competencies needed, 121, 122, 123–124
    DTRs in, 56, 120
    population-based focus of, 118, 119, 120,
        124, 125
    prevention of illness and levels of
        prevention, 120
    public health nutrition, 118–120
    research in, 219
    specialty areas of practice, 122–124, 123*t*
    supervised practice in, 43
Community colleges, 11. *See also*
    Coordinated Program in Dietetics (CP)
Community learning experiences, 204
Community service, 204
Compensation. *See* Salaries
Competencies. *See also* Standards of Practice
    (SOP)
    in dietetic practice, 27, 43, 54, 66
    future trends for, 235, 237, 240–241, 242
    of healthcare managers, 180–181, 180*f*
    of leaders, 111–112*t*, 168
    of managers, 110–111, 180–181, 180*f*
    multicultural, 246
    standards of professional performance, 56,
        66–67, 93–94, 109–111
The Competitive Edge (Helm), 139–140
Compulsive eating, 153–154
Conceptual skills in management, 178–180
Conflict management, 175
Consultant Dietitians in Health Care
    Facilities (DPG), 133
Consultants, 11, 12*t*, 127–142
    in business practice, 134–135
    characteristics of, 128
    contracts and fees, 130–131
    defined, 140
    ethical and legal bases of practice,
        139–140

in extended care, 53, 131–134
health care consultants, 131–134
mentors for, 128–129
personal liability, 68, 130
in private practice, 135–139, 137–139*t*,
    141
regulations governing, 132
standards for quality assurance, 133–134
standards of practice, 67
start-up, 128–131, 129–130*t*
Consumer education, 20, 113
Consumer message development model,
    202*f*, 204
Consumer surveys, 99, 204
Continuing education. *See also* Graduate
        education; Professional development
    for business and communications, 147
    for consultants in health and extended
        care, 131
    for consultants in private practice, 136,
        139
    for disordered eating specialists, 154
    importance of, 42, 237
    professional requirements, 9
    for registration and licensure, 47, 54, 60
Continuous quality improvement, 140
Contracts and fees of consultants, 130–131,
    134
Cooking schools, 5, 156
Cooper, Lenna Frances, 6, 7
Cooperative extension program, 118
Coordinated Program in Dietetics (CP), 38,
    41, 44, 48, 58
Correctional institutions. *See* Long-term care
Cost containment, 92, 175, 235
Counseling
    adherence counseling skills, 188
    in disordered eating, 153–154
    interviewing in, 198, 201*t*
    nutrition education and, 187
    patient-centered, 198–202, 201*t*
Credentialing, 10, 51–64. *See also* Licensure;
        Registration
    appropriate use of, 61
    CDR. *See* Commission on Dietetic
        Registration
    Certificates of Training, 59–60
    defined, 63

Credentialing (*Continued*)
  development of, 52–54
  dietetic technicians, 54
  DTR recertification, 54, 57, 60
  DTR registration, 11, 21, 55–58
  history of, 52
  legal regulation of dietitians and
    nutritionists, 61–62, 77–78
  RD examination, 54–55
  RD recertification, 54, 60
  specialist certification, 59
  specialist recertification, 60–61
Credential Registration and Maintenance
    System (CRMS), 58
Crimean War, 5
Cross-training, 139
CSG (Certified Specialist in Gerontological
    Nutrition), 59
CSO (Certified Specialist in Oncology
    Nutrition), 59
CSP (Certified Specialist in Pediatric
    Nutrition), 59
CSR (Certified Specialist in Renal
    Nutrition), 59
CSSD (Certified Specialist in Sports
    Dietetics), 59, 161
Culinary schools, 5, 156
Customer focus, 20

D
Data management, 72
Data management specialists, 123
Delivery of dietetic services, 214
Delivery of learning to dietetic professionals,
    71
Demographics, 226–227, 246
Designations, 10, 59, 61, 62. *See also*
    Credentialing; Licensure; Registration
Developmental diseases, 122–123, 132
Developmental disease specialist, 122
DHHS (Health and Human Services
    Department), 14, 18, 72, 78
Diabetes, 32, 67, 98, 147–148, 227
Diagnosis in nutrition care, 90, 120
"Dial-a-dietitian," 15
Didactic Program in Dietetics (DPD), 38,
    40–41, 48, 57
Diet and fitness industry, 235

Dietary Guidelines for Americans, 15, 78
Dietary Reference Intakes (DRIs), 235
Dietetic assistants, 98
Dietetic Practice Groups (DPGs), 27–31,
    28–30*t*
  in clinical nutrition management, 94
  Consultant Dietitians in Health Care
    Facilities, 133
  Dietitians in Business and
    Communications, 145
  Dietitians in Health Care Communities,
    133
  in education, 159, 160*t*
  in food and nutrition systems
    management, 105
  history of, 12
  membership in, 22
  Nutrition Entrepreneurs, 134
  in research, 159, 160*t,* 215
  Sports, Cardiovascular and Wellness
    Nutritionists, 148
  sub-units of, 259–261
Dietetics. *See* American Dietetic Association
    (ADA); Profession of dietetics
Dietetics Community (ADA's social
    network), 232
Dietetics Practice-Based Research Network,
    212
Dietetic Technician Program (DT), 11, 41,
    44, 57–58
Dietetic Technicians, Registered (DTR),
    55–58
  areas of practice, 55–57, 95–98
  Certificates of Training, 59–60
  in clinical practice, 95–98
  in community and public health
    nutrition, 56, 120
  credentialing of, 11, 21, 54, 55–58
  defined, 17
  Dietetic Technician Program, 11, 41, 55,
    57–58
  educational roles of, 187
  education requirements for, 11, 38
  in extended care, 133
  in food and nutrition systems
    management, 56
  "Future Practice and Education" Task
    Force, 13, 42, 56

on healthcare teams, 55, 56, 57, 95, 110
licensure in Maine, 55, 61
as managers, 104–105
median wage for, 46
membership in ADA, 21
recertification, 57, 60
registration, 27, 57–58
relationship with RDs, 56–57
requirements for, 11
responsibilities of, 57
specialties of practice, 56–57
standards, 56
as supervisors, 104–105
Web sites, 58
Dietetic Technicians, Registered (DTRs)
employment settings, 87*t*
Dietitians, defined, 4, 52, 86
Dietitians in Business and Communications
(DPG), 145
Dietitians in Health Care Communities
(DPG), 133
"Dietitian's Week" observance, 15
Diet therapy, 7, 86, 101. *See also* Clinical
nutrition; Medical nutritional
therapists (MNTs)
The Directory of Dietetics Programs (ADA),
43, 47
Disordered eating, 148, 150, 153–154,
161
Distance learning, 69, 71, 147
Diversity, 174, 227, 228–230*t*, 231, 241
Doctor of Education (EdD) degrees, 45
Doctor of Philosophy (PhD) degrees, 45
Domain of learning, 208
DPD. *See* Didactic Program in Dietetics
DPGs. *See* Dietetic Practice Groups
DRIs (Dietary Reference Intakes), 235
DT. *See* Dietetic Technician Program
DTRs. *See* Dietetic Technicians, Registered

E
Early practice of dietetics, 5–6
Eating disorders. *See* Disordered eating
EBP. *See* Evidence-based practice
Education of dietetic professional, 11, 12*t*,
37–49. *See also* Accreditation;
Continuing education; Graduate
education; Professional development

ADA examination requirements, 55
advanced-level, 44–48, 46*t*
allied health professionals compared, 237,
238*t*
in community and public health
nutrition, 122
continuing education, 9, 42, 44
Coordinated Program in Dietetics (CP),
38, 40–41, 44, 48
defined, 208
Didactic Program in Dietetics (DPD), 38,
40–41, 48, 57
dietetics requirements, 39–40
Dietetic Technician Program (DT), 11,
38, 41, 55, 57–58
distance learning, 69, 71, 147
financial aid, 10, 31–32, 43, 47
foundation knowledge and competencies,
8–9, 40
"Future Practice and Education" Task
Force, 13, 42, 56
graduate program experience, 47
internships, 38, 40–41, 43–44
"Master Plan for Education and Practice"
(ADA), 13
outcome-based, 9, 38, 39, 189, 195
program requirements, 38–39
RD requirements, 55
researcher preparation, 159
research experience, 47–48
self-responsibility for, 72–74, 73*t*, 74*t*
for sports nutrition, 150–151
"Standards of Education," 9
supervised practice, 38, 39, 40, 41,
43–44, 48, 57–58
technology in, 71
trends, 41–43
undergraduate programs, 38–39, 40–41,
48, 57, 145
Educators, dietitians as, 154–158, 185–210
adults as learners, 205–206
assessment instruments, 191–192
assessment of needs of learners, 189
as coaches, 197
in colleges and universities, 156
as communicators, 202–204, 202*f*, 203*f*
in community colleges, 156
as counselors, 189–202, 201*t*

Educators, dietitians as (*Continued*)
  designing instruction, 189–195
  in elementary and secondary schools, 155
  evaluation of educational program, 195
  in industry-based education, 157–158
  instructional design model, use of, 195
  instructional methods, 194–195
  instructional strategy, 192–194, 193*t*
  learning to teach, 187–189, 188*t*
  in medical and dental education,
    156–157
  mentoring. *See* Mentoring
  in nursing and allied health education,
    157
  performance objectives, 189–191
  practice groups for, 159, 160*t*
  as preceptors, 197–198, 199–200*t*
  roles of educators, 196–204
  teaching groups and teams, 206–207
  teaching skills, 186, 187–188, 188*t*
  theories of learning, 188
  types of learning, 189, 204–205
  in worksite nutrition education, 158
Elderly adults, 152, 203*f*, 204, 226–227,
    228–230*t*, 231, 240
Electronic communications security, 69
Electronic health records, 72, 100, 232
The Entrepreneurial Nutritionist (Helm),
    128, 131
Entrepreneurs, 128, 134, 135, 136, 149,
    241, 243
Environmental health and food safety
    specialists, 123
Environmental issues, 233–234
Epigenetics, 234–235, 234*f*
Ethics, 67–69, 139–140
  "Code of Ethics for the Profession of
    Dietetics and Process for Consideration
    of Ethical Issues," 9, 57, 69, 249–251
  of consultants, 68*t*, 132–133, 139–140
  defined, 79
  management and, 179
Ethnic diversity, 226, 227
Evaluation
  of educational program, 195
  nutrition care process and model, 92
Evidence Analysis Library (ADAF), 32, 75,
    93, 215, 217

Evidence-based practice (EBP), 40, 75–76,
    76–77*t*, 79, 92–93, 215–217, 221
Examination requirements for RDs, 10,
    54–55, 58
Extended care consultants, 53, 131–134
Extended care facilities, 94, 101, 128, 131,
    132. *See also* Long-term care

F
FANSA (Food and Nutrition Science
    Alliance), 14
Fast food, 42, 227, 231
Fats, 4
FDA. *See* Food and Drug Administration
Federal regulation. *See* Regulation
Fees for consulting, 130–131
"Fellow of the American Dietetic
    Association," 59
Financial aid, 10, 31–32, 43, 47
Fitness, 147, 150, 235. *See also* Sports
    nutrition; Wellness and health
    promotion
Food and Culinary Professionals (DPG), 105
Food and Drug Administration (FDA), 78,
    104, 217
Food and food service industries, 158, 218,
    235, 237, 242
Food and nutrition. *See also* Food and
    nutrition systems management
  advanced degrees in, 47
  attitudes toward, 227, 228–230*t*, 231
Food and Nutrition Board, 15
Food and Nutrition Conference and
    Exposition (FNCE), 69
Food and Nutrition Science Alliance
    (FANSA), 14
Food and nutrition systems management, 7,
    103–115
  in acute care, 105–106
  as area of practice, 11, 12*t*
  career path in, 108, 112–113, 242–243
  in commercial food services, 108–109
  dietetic practice groups in, 105
  employment areas, 104–109
  in healthcare facilities, 108
  history of, 104
  in hospitality and retail food services,
    108–109

industry reengineering, 237
leadership competencies, 111, 111–112*t*
in long-term care, 106–107
management standards, 110–111
in noninstitutional settings, 107
production and service systems, 106
salaries in, 105
in school nutrition programs, 107–108
specialties of practice, 124
standards of practice, 109–112
supervised practice in, 43
Food conservation programs, 6
Food managers in AMFO, 10–11
Food Marketing Institute, 144
Food production, 106, 113, 243. *See also*
Food and nutrition systems
management
Food safety and sanitation, 56, 78, 110,
123–124, 144, 235
Food science research, 214
Food service administration, 11. *See also*
Food and nutrition systems
management
Food services, defined, 113
"Foundation Knowledge and Competencies"
(CADE), 40
Frances Stern Clinic, 5
Future of dietetics, 42, 56, 225–248
age diversity and, 227
aging population in, 231
changing demographics, 226–227
changing roles in healthcare systems,
235–236
communication technology in, 232–233
competencies, 237, 240–241
competencies of dietetics professionals in,
238*t*
competition and collaboration, 239–240
environmental issues in, 233–234
ethnic diversity and, 227
food and food service industries, 242–243
health and wellness in, 231–232
implications and challenges for, 236–239
information technology and management,
243
lifelong learning and, 237
nutrigenomics and nanotechnology,
234–235

planning for, 244–246
public service and military, 244
reengineering, 237
research, 243–244
roles for professionals in, 241–242
"Future Practice and Education" Task Force
(ADA), 13, 42, 56

G
General clinical research centers (GCRCs),
217–218
Generalist vs. specialist dietitians, 53
Generational diversity, 174, 227–231,
228–230*t*
Generation X, 228–230*t*
Genetics, 234–235, 234*f*
Gen Y, 228–230*t*
Gerontological Nutrition, Certified
Specialist in (CSG), 59
Goal setting, 60, 170, 171, 178–179
Governmental agencies, 14–15, 77–78, 128,
131, 244. *See also* Community and
public health nutrition; *specific agencies*
Governmental regulation. *See* Regulation
Government-sponsored centers and
laboratories, 218–219
Graduate education, 44–48. *See also*
Continuing education
business exposure in, 145
for educators and researchers, 159
future challenges and, 237
for sports nutrition, 150
Graves, Lulu Grace, 6, 7

H
Harvard Business Review as interpersonal
skills resource, 174
Headquarters organization chart (ADA), 24,
258
Health agencies, 118, 119, 121. *See also*
Governmental agencies
Health and Human Services Department
(DHHS), 14, 18, 72, 78
Health and wellness. *See* Wellness and health
promotion
Health care accessibility, 226, 236
Health care consultants, 131–134. *See also*
Consultants

Healthcare costs, 213, 235

Healthcare engineering, 237–238

Healthcare facilities

clinical nutrition management in, 108

dietetics in early, 5

regulation of consultants in, 131, 132

Healthcare Leadership Alliance, 180, 180*f*

Healthcare market, 226–227, 236–237

Healthcare reform, 11, 92, 98–99, 235–236

Healthcare system, changes in, 124, 226

Healthcare teams. *See* Teams in healthcare

Health Insurance Portability and Accountability Act of 1996 (HIPAA), 132

Health promotion. *See* Wellness and health promotion

Healthy Eating Index, 78

"Healthy People 2010," 16, 242

Heart disease, 147–148, 151, 161

High blood pressure, 147–148

HIPAA (Health Insurance Portability and Accountability Act of 1996), 132

Historical milestones of profession of dietetics, 9–15

Home health specialists, 124, 132

Hospital, Institution, and Educational Food Service Society (HIEFSS), 10

Hospitality food services, 108–109, 156. *See also* Food and nutrition systems management

Hospitals, 5, 108. *See also* Healthcare facilities

House of Delegates (ADA), 25–26

Huddleston, Mary P., 8

Human relations skills in management, 174–178

Human resources, defined, 113

Human services, 118, 119

Hypertension, 147–148

I

Industry-based education, 157–158

Influential leaders of profession of dietetics, 7–8

Informatics, 72, 233

Information technology, 233, 238, 239–240, 243. *See also* Technology

Innovation, 20

Inpatient care, 94–95, 97–98, 108, 128. *See also* Clinical nutrition

Institutional food service management, 107, 109. *See also* Food and nutrition systems management

Instruction, defined, 208

Insurance for personal liability, 75, 130

Integrated health systems, 235

Integrity, 20. *See also* Ethics

Interdisciplinary teams, 121, 151, 153–154, 235

International career opportunities, 244

International Confederation of Dietetic Associations, 15

International Congress of Dietetics, 15

Internships, 38, 40–41, 43–44, 145, 204, 205

Interpersonal relationships skills, 174, 182, 188, 241

Intervention in nutrition care, 90, 120

Interviewing in counseling, 198, 201*t*

Intrapreneurs, 137, 140

J

Job skills in management, 175

Joint Commission on Accreditation of Healthcare Organizations (JCAHO), 78

Journal of the American Dietetic Association, 7, 22, 53, 220

K

The Knowledge Executive (Cleveland), 240

L

Latinos, 227

Lawsuits, 74–75

Leadership, 167–170, 171–172*t*

competencies, 111–112*t*

defined, 182

of early dietetics, 7–8

in food and nutrition management, 111, 111–112*t*

future trends, 240

management vs., 166*t*, 167

quality and efficiency improvements through, 169, 169–170*t*

transformative, 111–112, 144
Leadership in Dietetics: Achieving a Vision for the Future (Barker, Arensberg, & Schiller), 167
Learning
adults as learners, 205–206
theories of, 188
types of, 204–205
Legal basis of practice, 74–75, 100, 139–140. *See also* Accreditation; Ethics; Licensure; Registration
Legal regulation of dietitians and nutritionists, 61–62
Legislative activity (ADA), 11, 32, 78
Liability, 74–75
Licensed Dietitians (LDs), 10, 17
Licensure, 10, 61–62. *See also* Credentialing; Registration
continuing education and, 47
of dietetic technicians in Maine, 55, 61
of dietitians, 47, 61–62, 77–78
of DTRs, 55
licensing, defined, 63
Task Force, 13
Lifelong professional development, 69–74. *See also* Continuing education; Professional development
Lobbying, 11
Long-range planning, 12–13, 170, 244–246
Long-term care. *See also* Clinical nutrition
clinical practice in, 87
consultants, 53, 131–134
defined, 140
extended care facilities, 94, 101, 128, 131, 132
federal and state regulation of, 106–107
food and nutrition management in, 106–107

M
Maine licensure of dietetic technicians, 55, 61
Malnutrition, 86, 95, 97, 119
Malpractice, 74–75
Managed care, 140, 235
Management, 10–11, 170–182. *See also* Food and nutrition systems management
benchmarking, 176
change management, 179–180
in clinical nutrition, 88, 89*f,* 94, 108
coaching and mentoring, 174–175
communications, 174
in community and public health nutrition, 122, 123*t*
competencies of, 110–111, 180–181, 180*f*
conceptual skills, 173*f,* 178–180
conflict resolution, 175
defined, 104, 113, 170, 182
ethical conduct, 179
in extended care, 133
financial, 175–176
functions, 166, 170–171, 171–172*t*
human relations skills, 173*f,* 174–175
interpersonal relationships, 174
leadership vs., 166*t,* 167
manager, defined, 104
middle management skills, 173
networking, 175
of quality, 177–178
resource management, 175–176, 182
responsibilities, 166
roles (Mintzberg's), 171–172*t,* 181*t,* 182
skills and abilities of, 173–182, 173*f*
"soft skills," 166–167
standards of practice, 110–111
strategic planning and goal setting, 178–179, 183
team building, 177
technical skills, 173*f,* 175–178
technology know-how, 176–177
training and staff development, 176
Marketing, 110, 113, 147, 243
Mary Schwartz Rose Fellowship, 8
Master of Science (MS) degrees, 45, 47
"Master Plan for Education and Practice," 13
Maternal and child health, 11, 120, 123
Media, 233
Medicaid, 131
Medical and dental education, 156–157
Medical nutritional therapists (MNTs), 7, 61, 92–93. *See also* Clinical nutrition
Medical nutrition education, 220
Medicare, 32, 131

Medicare Medical Nutrition Therapy Act of 2007, 32
Member Interest Groups (MIGs), 10–11, 27–30, 261
Membership categories (ADA), 21–22, 47, 253–255
Membership in ADA, 9–10, 24, 43, 47, 52, 253–255
Mentoring
  in business and communications, 146
  for consultants, 128–129, 136–137
  defined, 182, 196
  educators as, 196–197
  managers as mentors, 174–175
Metabolic nutrition care, 59
Metabolomics, 234, 234f
Military, 6, 11, 244
Mintzberg's 10 managerial roles, 171–172t, 181t, 182
MNTs. See Medical nutritional therapists
Monitoring and evaluation in nutrition care process, 92
Motivational interviewing, 198
MS (Master of Science) degrees, 45, 47
Multicultural competencies, 241, 246
Multidisciplinary roles, 239, 246
Multidisciplinary teams, 121, 151, 153–154, 235
MyPyramid, 78

N
Nanotechnology, 234–235
National Academy of Sciences, 78, 244
National Food Service Management Institute, 108
National Health and Nutrition Examination Survey (NHANES III), 148
National Institutes of Health (NIH), 217, 242
National Nutrition Month, 15, 154–155
National School Lunch Act of 1966, 11
Native Americans, 118
NCPM (Nutrition care process and model), 90–92, 91f, 93–94
Nebraska, medical nutrition therapists in, 61
Needs assessment in food and nutrition services, 133
Networking, 71, 136, 146, 161, 175, 232

New York Cooking Academy, 5
NHANES III (National Health and Nutrition Examination Survey), 148
Niacin, 5
Nightingale, Florence, 5
NIH (National Institutes of Health), 217, 242
Noninstitutional food service management, 107, 109. See also Food and nutrition systems management
Nontraditional careers, 134, 135, 144, 146, 161
Nursing and allied health, 157
Nursing care consultants, 53, 131–134
Nursing homes. See Clinical nutrition; Long-term care
Nutrient delivery systems, 235
Nutrigenomics, 234–235, 234f
Nutrition assessment. See Assessment
Nutrition care process and model (NCPM), 90–92, 91f, 93–94
Nutrition care standards of practice, 93–94
Nutrition Entrepreneurs (DPG), 134, 197
Nutrition Foundation, 15
Nutrition Information Work Group, 72
Nutritionist, defined, 17
Nutrition-related disorders, 234
Nutrition screening, 133, 141

O
Obesity
  in children, 148, 150, 153, 232
  as eating disorder, 153
Office of the Surgeon General, 6
Older adults. See Aging population
Omnibus Reconciliation Act of 1987, 131
Oncology Nutrition, Certified Specialist in (CSO), 59
Open-ended questioning, 198, 201t
Organizational awareness, 241
Osteoporosis, 147–148
Outcomes research, 217, 221
Outpatient and ambulatory care, 94, 101, 128

P
Part-time employment, 131–132, 135–136
Patient-centered counseling, 198, 202

Patients' rights, 132
PBL (Problem-based learning), 157, 204–205
Pediatric Nutrition, Certified Specialist in (CSP), 59
Pellagra, 5
"Performance, Proficiency, and Value Plan" (ADA), 70
Performance standards in dietetics, 56, 66–67, 93–94, 109–111
Personal focus in community nutrition, 118, 120, 124
Personal liability insurance, 75, 130
Pew Health Professions Commission recommendations, 235–236
Pharmaceuticals, 134, 144, 151
Physiology and nutrition research, 214
Plato, 8
Political action committee, 11
Population-based focus of community and public health nutrition, 125–126
Position papers (ADA), 16, 30–31, 148–149, 263–267
Practice-Based Research Network, 212
Practitioner, defined, 63
Preceptors, 48, 154, 197–198, 199–200*t*. *See also* Supervised practice
Prescriptive authority in clinical practice, 100
Presentation skills, 188
Prevention of illness
  by allied health professionals, 157
  community nutrition dietitians, 120
  developmental diseases and, 122–123
  wellness and fitness programs and, 147–148
  worksite fitness programs and, 151, 152, 231
Privacy procedures, 132
Private practice consultants, 11, 12*t*, 135–139, 137–139*t*
Privileging, 100
Problem-based learning (PBL), 157, 204–205
Problem-definition skills, 241
Problem-solving skills, 241
Product safety, 144
Profession, defined, 8, 79

Professional, defined, 17
Professional areas of practice. *See* Areas of practice
Professional Code of Ethics, 9, 57, 69, 249–251. *See also* Ethics
Professional development, 69–74. *See also* Continuing education; Education of dietetic professional
  certification and, 70–71
  compensation improvement through, 69–70
  delivery of learning in, 71
  distance learning, 69, 71, 147
  lifelong learning and, 70–71
  management's role in, 174–175, 176
  portfolio, 60–61, 65, 70–71, 178
  as preparation for future, 245–246
  self-responsibility for learning in, 72–74, 73*t*, 74*t*
Professional Development Portfolio (PDP), 60, 70–71
Professional Development Resource Center (ADA), 70
Professional partnerships, 14–15
Professional performance responsibilities, 70
Professional practice, 65–82. *See also* Credentialing; Professional development; Registration
  certification, 53, 59–61, 62, 70–71
  communication standards of, 109
  competencies of future professionals, 235, 240–241, 242
  defined, 17
  delivery of learning, 71
  ethics, 9, 57, 67–69, 68*t*, 79
  evidence-based practice, 40, 75–76, 76–77*t*, 79
  future challenges, 236–239. *See also* Future of dietetics
  future roles in, 241–246
  government influence in, 77–78
  history of, 8–9
  informatics, 72
  legal basis of, 74–75
  licensure, 10, 13, 47, 55, 61–62, 63, 66
  lifelong development, 69–74
  model of, 66

Professional practice (*Continued*)
  "The Profession of Dietetics: The Report
    of the Study Commission on
    Dietetics," 13
  scope of, 66–67
  self-responsibility for learning, 72–74,
    73*t*, 74*t*
  standards of, 40, 52, 66–67
Profession of dietetics
  ADA. *See* American Dietetic Association
  ADAF. *See* American Dietetic Association
    Foundation
  areas of practice, 11–12, 12*t*
  clinics, 5
  cooking schools, 5
  dietetic practice groups, 12
  dietetic technicians and managers, 10–11
  early practice of, 5–6
  growth and historical milestones, 9–15
  history of, 3–18
  hospital dietetics, 5
  influential leaders, 7–8
  legislative activity, 11, 32, 78
  long-range planning, 12–13, 244–246
  membership, 9–10
  military, 6
  overview, 8–9
  professional partnerships, 14–15
  public outreach, 15–16, 52, 99–100,
    121–122
  registration and licensure, 10
"The Profession of Dietetics: The Report of
  the Study Commission on Dietetics,"
  13
Program planning, defined, 126
Project-based learning, 205
Proteonomics, 234, 234*f*
Psychomotor skills, defined, 208
Public health, 118–119, 120, 122–124. *See
  also* Community and public health
  nutrition
  dietetic knowledge and, 52, 66
Public Health Service (USPHS), 14
Public opinion surveys on clinical practice,
  99
Public outreach
  by ADA, 9, 13
  in clinical practice, 99–100

  in community and public health
    nutrition, 121–122
  early concern for, 52
  educational activities in, 187
  history of, 15–16
Public policy, 78, 79
Public service, 244

Q
Quality assurance program, 134, 136, 178
Quality improvement
  continuous, 140
  leadership for, 169, 169–170*t*
Quality management, 177–178
Quality Management Committee (ADA),
  90, 177–178

R
RDs. *See* Registered Dietitians
Recertification, 54, 57, 60–61
Recycling, 233
Red Cross, 5, 6
Reengineering, 237
Registered Dietitians (RDs), 10, 27, 42, 44.
    See also specific areas of practice
  Certificates of Training, 59–60
  certification title, 53
  as community nutrition resource, 121
  continuing education, 42, 54
  credentialing, 42–43, 54–55, 61–62
  defined, 17
  designation from CDR, 27
  education, 39–40, 42–43
  educational activities of, 186–187
  employment settings, 87*t*, 88*t*
  examination, 54–55
  financial advantages of advanced
    education, 46–47
  as managers, 104–105
  recertification, 54, 60
  relationship with DTR, 56–57
  state regulation of, 61–62
  supervised practice, 43–44
  as supervisors, 104–105
Registration, 10, 53–58. *See also*
    Certification; Commission on
    Dietetic Registration; Credentialing;
    Licensure

defined, 62
DTRs, 55–58
RDs, 10, 54–55
Regulation
   of dietitians and nutritionists, 61–62
   of extended care facilities, 106–107, 128, 131–132
   of healthcare, 77–78, 79
   of health care facilities, 128, 131–132
Reimbursement of services, 32, 75, 98, 130–131
Renal disease, 32, 98
Renal Nutrition, Certified Specialist in (CSR), 59
Research, 155, 158–160, 211–222
   in academic health centers, 217–218
   ADA philosophy on, 213
   ADA Research Committee, 213–215
   applications, 215–217, 216f
   applied studies, 159, 212
   areas of practice, 12t, 158–159, 214, 217–220
   in cardiovascular nutrition, 151
   career opportunities in, 158–159, 217–220
   clinical studies, 159
   committee of the ADA, 213–215
   in community and public health, 219
   in controlled working environments, 159, 212
   defined, 221
   Dietetics Practice-Based Research Network, 212
   dietitians in, 158–159, 160t
   DPG, 215
   evidence analysis process, 215–217
   experience in graduate studies, 47–48
   in food and industry companies, 218
   funding, 31–32, 215, 217, 220
   future trends, 243–244
   in general clinical research centers, 217–218
   in government centers and laboratories, 218–219
   in graduate studies, 47–48
   importance of, 212–213
   in laboratories, 158–159, 212
   in lipid research clinics, 151
   in nutrition research centers, 215, 219–220
   outcomes research, 217, 221
   practice groups, 159, 160t, 215
Research: Successful Approaches (Monsen & Van Horn), 213
Resource allocation, defined, 114
Resource management, 175–176, 182
Restaurants and retail food services, 108–109. *See also* Food and food service industries
Richards, Ellen H., 7
Roberts, Lydia J., 8
Rorer, Sarah Tyson, 7
Rose, Mary Schwartz, 8
Rural practice, 55, 132, 226

S
Safety in products, 144
Salaries
   ADA efforts to increase, 69–70
   of dietetic professionals, 22–24, 23t, 46, 46t, 105
   Dietetics Compensation and Benefits Survey, 45, 128
   education level and, 46, 46t, 69–70
   equity and trends, 238–239
   in food and nutrition systems management, 105
SCAN (Sports and Cardiovascular Nutritionists), a DPG, 148
School-based health centers, 155
School nutrition, 11, 107–108, 155
School Nutrition Association, 108
School Nutrition Services (DPG), 108
"The Scope of Dietetic Practice" framework, 10, 55, 62, 66
Scope of practice, 63, 66–67, 177–178
Scurvy, 4–5
Security, 58, 69
Self-responsibility for learning, 72–74, 73t, 74t
Service learning, 204
Services, defined, 101
Service teams in clinical nutrition, 88, 89f, 94–98
Shared decision-making, 76
Short-term medical treatment, 105–106

Silent Generation (born before 1945), 228–230*t*

Site visits (CADE), 39

Smith, Florence, 52

SNAP (Supplemental Nutrition Assistance Program), 78

Social networks, 71, 232

Social responsibility, 20

Social welfare dietetics, 7. *See also* Community and public health nutrition

"Soft skills" of managers, 166

SOP. *See* Standards of practice

SOPP. *See* Standards of Professional Performance

Specialist certification, 59
  recertification, 60–61

Specialist vs. generalist dietitians, 53

Special Supplemental Nutrition Program for Women, Infants and Children (WIC), 78, 120

Specialties of practice. *See also* Dietetic Practice Groups (DPGs); *specific areas of practice*
  board-certified, 59
  in chronic disease prevention and control, 122
  in clinical nutrition, 95
  in community and public health nutrition, 122–124, 123*t*
  in disordered eating, 148, 150, 153–154
  for DTRs, 56–57
  generalist vs. specialist, 52–53
  in genetic dietetics, 234–235
  information specialists, 243
  nutrition intervention, 243
  specialty, defined, 59
  standards developed for, 67

"Spokesperson network," 15

Sports, Cardiovascular and Wellness Nutritionists (SCAN), 148

Sports Dietetics, Certified Specialist in (CSSD), 59, 161

Sports nutrition, 148–151, 149*t*
  American College of Sports Medicine Exercise Test Technology certification, 139

defined, 161

Standards for quality assurance, 133–134

Standards of practice (SOP), 66–67
  application of knowledge, 109
  clinical nutrition, 93–94
  in communication, 109
  in consultation, 67
  for DTRs, 56
  for extended care consultants, 133–134
  general, 110
  for health care consultants, 133–134
  in management, 110
  in nutrigenomics, 234
  in nutrition care, 93–94
  quality in practice, 109
  in utilization and management of resources, 109

Standards of Professional Performance (SOPP), 56, 66–67, 93–94, 109–111

Starting practice, 136–137, 146

State and district associations (ADA), 31

State departments of health, 132

State regulation. *See* Licensure; Regulation

Statutory certification, 61–62

Strategic plan (ADA), 13, 20–21, 33

Strategic planning, 178–179, 183

Strokes, 147–148

Student teaching, 47

Subacute care, 141

Sub-units of Dietetic Practice Groups (DPGs) and Member Interest Groups (MIGs), 27, 259–261

Summative evaluation, 195

Supervised practice, 43–44, 48
  in coordinated program in dietetics, 41
  defined, 48
  for DTRs, 43–44, 57–58
  for DTs, 41, 57–58
  RD preceptor, 43, 48
  for RDs, 38, 39, 40, 43–44, 55

Supervision, defined, 208

Supervisor skills, 173, 173*f*

Supplemental Nutrition Assistance Program (SNAP), 78

Supplemental Nutrition Program for Women, Infants, and Children (WIC), 78, 120

Surgeon General's Office, 6
Synchronous technologies in distance
    learning, 71

T
Task Forces (ADA)
    "Future Practice and Education," 13, 42,
    56
    Health Care Reform Task Group,
    98–99
    for long-range planning, 13
Teaching, 189–195, 193*t*. *See also*
    Educators, dietitians as
Teams in healthcare
    clinical service teams, 88, 89*f,* 94–98
    defined, 125
    DTRs' role on, 55, 56, 57, 95, 110
    multidisciplinary, 121, 151, 153–154,
    235, 245
    teaching of, 206–207
    team building skills, 176, 177, 241
    training, 176
Technical skills in management, 175–178
Technicians, dietetic. *See* Dietetic
    Technicians, Registered (DTR)
Technology
    communication trends, 232–233
    educational, 71
    electronic communications security, 69
    electronic health records, 72, 100
    healthcare engineering, 237–238
    informatics, 72
    information management, future roles,
    243
    job performance benefits, 176–177
    legal issues of, 74
    in management, 176–177
    in professional development, 71
Telehealth, 9, 74, 99–100, 232
Terminology, 74, 92
Tertiary prevention of illnesses, 120
Therapeutic dietitians. *See* Clinical nutrition
Titles permitted, 10, 59, 61, 62. *See also*
    Credentialing; Licensure; Registration
Training. *See also* Education of dietetic
    professional; Educators, dietitians as
    defined, 208

in-service sessions, 133
in technology, 177
Transformative leadership, 111–112, 144
Treatise on Scurvy (Lind), 4
Trends. *See* Future of dietetics
*Trends—Consumer Attitudes and the
    Supermarket* (Food Marketing
    Institute), 144
"Two by two" program, 38, 41, 44, 48

U
Undergraduate education, 38–39, 40–41,
    48, 57, 145
Underserved groups' health care access, 119,
    226
Universities and colleges, 107, 156,
    217–218. *See also* Education of dietetic
    professional; Graduate education
U.S. Dietary Guidelines for Americans, 15,
    78
U.S. Public Health Service (USPHS), 14
USDA (U.S. Department of Agriculture),
    78
Utilization and management of resources
    standards of professional practice, 109

V
Value system, 161, 190
The Venture (Research DPG), 215
Veteran's Administration, 11
Video instruction, 71
Vitamins and minerals, 4, 5

W
Web sites, 15, 55, 58, 71, 147, 153
Weight management certification programs,
    59–60, 155
Wellness and health promotion, 147–154
    allied health professionals and, 157
    areas of practice, 148, 151–152
    cardiovascular nutrition, 151
    competencies in, 152
    disordered eating, 153–154
    future of, 231–232
    health promotion, defined, 161
    information for, 152–153
    private practice in, 151

Wellness and health promotion (*Continued*)
   sports nutrition, 148–151, 149*t*
   Web sites for, 153
   wellness, defined, 161
   worksite programs for, 151, 152
Wheeler, Ruth, 8
Women
   in business, 135, 226
   as learners, 194

   maternal and infant health, 11, 123
   salary equity for, 238–239
   women's health, 16, 124
Women, Infants, and Children Program
   (WIC), 78, 120, 132
Worksite wellness programs, 151, 152
World War I, 6, 11
World War II, 6